RADIANT BRIDE

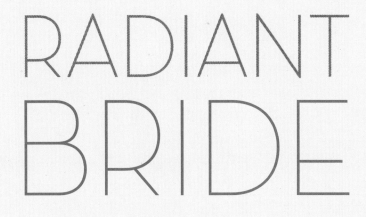

The Beauty, Diet, Fitness, and Fashion Plan for Your Big Day

◁ ALEXIS WOLFER ▷

RUNNING PRESS
PHILADELPHIA · LONDON

Published by Running Press,
A Member of the Perseus Books Group
All rights reserved under the Pan-American and International Copyright Conventions

Printed in China

Books published by Running Press are available at special discounts for bulk purchases in the United States by corporations, institutions, and other organizations. For more information, please contact the Special Markets Department at the Perseus Books Group, 2300 Chestnut Street, Suite 200, Philadelphia, PA 19103, or call (800) 810-4145, ext. 5000, or e-mail special.markets@perseusbooks.com.

ISBN 978-0-7624-5748-9
Library of Congress Control Number: 2015935931

E-book ISBN 978-0-7624-5809-7

9 8 7 6 5 4 3 2 1
Digit on the right indicates the number of this printing

Edited by Cindy De La Hoz
Designed by Susan Van Horn
Illustrations by Tracy Turnbull
Illustrations on pages 52-57, 87, and 91 by Susan Van Horn
Typography: Great Vibes, Neutra, and Port Ornaments

Running Press Book Publishers
2300 Chestnut Street
Philadelphia, PA 19103-4371

Visit us on the web!
www.runningpress.com

For the most radiant bride and groom I know:
my mom and dad.
You make fifty-plus years of wedded bliss
seem like a piece of cake.

❧ CONTENTS ❧

GUIDELINES

Before you embark on your *Radiant Bride* journey, here are some mostly common sense guidelines to keep in mind.

1) You know your body best. Listen to it. If something doesn't feel right (whether it's a new fitness move, skincare tip, or anything else), skip it.

2) Your health and wellness are always my number-one priority. Pretty please, talk with a doctor before starting any type of new fitness routine or diet.

3) Don't eat anything or use anything topically that contains any ingredients you're allergic to.

4) If anything new you use topically (a new DIY facial, for example) irritates your skin in any way, rinse it off immediately and seek medical attention if symptoms persist.

5) As with anything, you get what you give. Give your best and I promise you will look and feel your best when your wedding day arrives.

6) Stand up straight and smile! Okay, so those aren't guidelines for using this book, per se, but they are my two absolute best tips for looking radiant, so we may as well get started with them now!

YOU SAID YES!

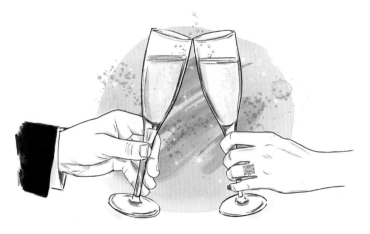

HI THERE, BEAUTIFUL BRIDES-TO-BE!

If I know one thing, it's that every woman wants to look and feel *amazing* on her wedding day. They want skin that glows, hair that shines, and a body that rocks. But far too many women are going about it all wrong—and it's backfiring. From crash-dieting and crazy fitness fads that leave brides' hair falling out, skin dull and drab, and energy levels in the gutter; to poor beauty choices, like scheduling a last-minute facial, rocking red nail polish, or getting a spray tan (more on all these later!), it's no wonder that, come wedding day, so many brides look and feel far from their radiant selves. And, well, I'm here to fix all that!

The most common question I get from readers of TheBeautyBean.com, is related to their upcoming nuptials. From what diet they should follow and when they should get their hair colored to tips on how to pick the most flattering dress and pose perfectly in pictures, brides want to know it all. *You* want to know it all! (It's why you picked up this book, isn't it?)

As I started receiving more and more e-mails, tweets, and Facebook messages, I knew I needed to find a solution. At first, I tried tracking down the best wedding bloggers, with the hopes of directing all the desperate brides-to-be there, but came up short. Too many of them were merely telling other brides what they had done, what makeup they wore, how they styled their hair, but it failed to take into account the fact that not all of their readers have the same taste, budget, skin tone, hair texture or length, or any number of other factors in common. So, I hit up my local bookstore. I scoured the shelves thinking I would be able to find the ultimate guide for the soon-to-be-Mrs. but instead I found shelves lined with books designed to help you plan the perfect party (some with mention of your hair, makeup, and dress), but none designed just for you, the bride.

So, I did what I've always done when confronted with the realization that something necessary doesn't exist and that I'm uniquely qualified to create it: I DIY'd it—and now, beautiful ladies, it's in your hands.

As a longtime beauty editor, the creator of the popular online women's magazine TheBeautyBean.com, and a beauty expert (as seen on *Today*, *E! News*, *The Doctors*, and more), I know (almost!) all there is to know about makeup, skincare, and hair. As a certified holistic health coach, I know (almost!) everything you need to know about dieting for your big day and eating for beauty. And, with a "do-it-yourself" (or DIY) focus (it is, after all, why *Access Hollywood* named me the "Female Beauty MacGyver"), my goal is to always give you the tools so you can do it all yourself!

Here you have it: the only bridal book designed just for you, the bride.

In *Radiant Bride*, you'll find everything you need to know to radiate on your wedding day. In this book, you have access to me: your own customizable and personal nutritionist, trainer, fashion stylist, beauty expert, life coach, and more.

First up, you'll learn how to show off that sparkling new ring of yours and make your hands look their best. You know, so you can send the prettiest of pictures to your friends and family to share the good news. (Or just brag to your Facebook "friends.") Then, we'll tackle what I know all brides (or at least the vast majority) are concerned with: getting into fighting shape. To ensure you hit all your diet and fitness goals, I've created the Radiant Bride Detox + Diet, based on my practice as a holistic health coach, certified by the Institute for Integrative Nutrition. It starts with a twenty-one-day detox and ends with you knowing the best long-term diet for you. This isn't a cookie-cutter diet (because when was the last time you heard of a single diet that actually worked for everyone?!); it's an in-depth, fully personalized plan that is guaranteed to work unlike any other diet you've tried. And then, of course, we'll tone with my tried-and-tested workouts designed to get you the biggest bang for your buck, by targeting your workouts to the body parts you're showing off in the dress of your dreams. But don't worry, this won't be all work and no play. I will also show you how to party your heart out for your bachelorette without blowing your diet or looking and feeling like crap the next day.

And for when you head out dress shopping (with this book in tow!), I'll break down how to pick out the most flattering wedding-dress style and shade of white for your body and skin tone, so you can confidently strut down the aisle. And, of course, you'll also learn how to take care of your beauty routine—including the products you need to toss and the new ones you need for your specific skin type so you radiate from today until well past your wedding day.

But that's not all.

In the pages of this book, you'll also get access to all my insider tips to help you seamlessly schedule all your prenuptial appointments and all my industry secrets to ensure you can handle any last-minute beauty or fashion emergency. There's a whole chapter for grooms, too (the rest of the book, however, is just for the ladies). And when the big day's done, I won't leave you hanging. I have you covered for your honeymoon and your happily ever after, too! Bottom line: this is *the* book you need to ensure you (and not just your centerpieces) radiate on the wedding day.

So, soon-to-be-Mrs.: Let's get started!

Love,
Alexis

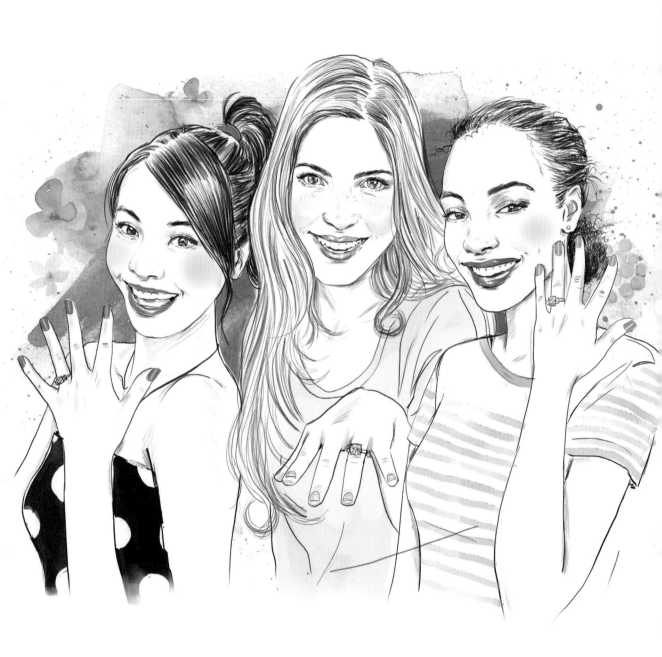

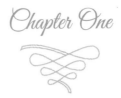

Chapter One

BLING, BLING: YOU'RE ENGAGED!

CONGRATULATIONS, LADY! You've landed the fiancé of your dreams and you're ready to tie the knot. But slow down, there's no need to rush. Sure, you've been planning your wedding since the ripe old age of five (when you saw your first Disney-princess movie, perhaps!) and are ready to get cranking on planning the wedding of the decade, but take a step back and enjoy your engagement for a bit. You just committed to spending your life with your soul mate. Relish in how special that is before jumping into the logistics of party planning. You'll only be engaged once; you'll be married forever, so enjoy it!

Whether you're anticipating your significant other popping the question or have already been engaged for a while, this chapter will give all you brides-to-be the tips you need to show off your new bling, brilliantly.

Research says 69 percent of you will have a professional engagement picture taken. My guess: 100 percent of you will be staging your own DIY photo shoot, including, of course, the ring selfie that you'll immediately send to your nearest and dearest.

Before you pull out that camera phone and start Instagramming pictures of that new rock of yours, it's time to get your hands in tip-top shape. You wouldn't pose for your wedding pictures without a swipe (or several) of makeup, and your engagement pictures (yes, even those that are just showing off your newly diamond-dipped digit) deserve a little TLC, too. No, I'm not referring to foundation and bronzer, but I am suggesting a bit of a hand facial, if you will, starting with a hydrating hand scrub and some manicure tips.

Quick Tip

Don't forget to call your VIPs before uploading your soon-to-be-perfect ring pic to Facebook. Your BFFs should know before those Facebook "friends" you haven't seen since middle school!

How to Get Your Hands in Picture-Perfect Shape

Off to get a manicure? Good for you! But before you do, use an exfoliating scrub at home. It will ensure the results of your salon stop or DIY mani (more on that below) are even better!

STEP 1

EXFOLIATE

DIY It . . .

Hands feeling dry and looking dull? This DIY Sugar + Honey Hand Healer will fix that. With raw honey, a natural moisturizer that's also antibacterial (to help protect your cuticles) and sugar to gently scrub away dry skin, this exfoliate is just what your hands need for their close-up. But please, do not use it if you have eczema, psoriasis, cuts, or a rash.

Sugar + Honey Hand Healer

3 tablespoons raw honey

1/4 cup white sugar

2 plastic bags

2 hair elastics

Mix the raw honey with the sugar until well combined. Apply generously to your hands, paying especially close attention to your cuticles. Cover each hand with one of the plastic bags, securing the bag around your wrist with the hair elastic. Let the hydrating scrub work its magic.

For deeper hydration, cover your plastic-wrapped hands in warm towels. After 15 minutes, wash your hands with your favorite facial cleanser (hand soaps can be too harsh). Pat your hands dry and follow with hand lotion (or a dab of coconut oil for an all-natural solution).

✃ *Quick Tips* ✃

Have some sunspots or discoloration you want to fade?
Add 2 tablespoons of lemon juice to your scrub. The citric acid acts like a gentle chemical peel, further helping to slough away those dark spots!

In a bind because your future-hubby just popped the question and your family/Twitter followers are pining for a pic?
Mix 2 tablespoons of white sugar with your favorite facial cleanser and vigorously wash your hands. Follow with moisturizer and, voilà!

Buy It . . .

Prefer to buy your hand scrub? Look for a sugar or nut-based scrub, not a salt scrub. In much the same way that salt dehydrates your body, a salt scrub pulls moisture from your skin when applied topically as well (and we most definitely don't want that!).

STEP 2

SHAPE + PAINT

Whether you're a weekly manicure kind of gal or more a "mani what?" woman, you're going to want your sparkler shots to really shine, and a lovely manicure will help to do just that. But not just for the reasons you think. Sure, a manicure will make your nails look especially gorgeous, elongate your fingers, and create the perfect canvas for making all your Facebook friends jealous, but the benefits far exceed that: it gives you a precious thirty minutes of "me time," which any bride-to-be knows is soon to be a hot commodity (what with all the food tastings, flower selecting, and dress fittings!).

Whether you go pro or DIY, here's what you need to know:

Nail Shape

The most flattering, elongating nail shapes are those that are slightly oval, giving the illusion of longer fingers, which will make your fingers appear leaner and your ring really pop. Sure, nail shape has to take into account your lifestyle (pointy talons won't last long if you type aggressively on a computer all day), but there are a few shapes that work well for all:

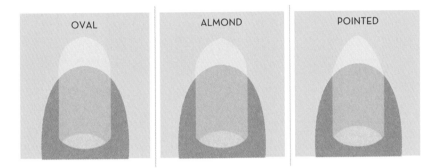

Try to avoid square nails, or at least round the corners. The blunt edge of a square nail shape draws the eye to the end, whereas more rounded nail shapes give the illusion of a longer nail.

Nail Color

Just as a nude heel helps to elongate your legs, the right nail polish color can similarly give the illusion of a longer finger (and a larger ring!). Sure, a bright hue is fun (feel free to rock it throughout the wedding planning process—if for no other reason than that it will make you smile when you look down at your candy-colored fingers), but when it's time to take the ring pics, it's highly recommended that you stick with a nude hue, which will vary based on your skin tone.

As a rule of thumb when picking a polish, look for a hue that, in the bottle, appears a shade or two lighter than your skin tone. Polish dries a bit darker than it appears in the bottle and you want your finished manicure to be just a touch lighter than your skin tone. Also, look for a shade with a pink undertone, which is universally flattering.

Sheer vs. Opaque

If you're going to DIY your manicure, sheer polishes are much more forgiving if you mess up—and conceal chips (should they happen), too! But, beware of the condition of your natural nail bed. If you have any discolorations, they'll show through.

~ Quick Tip ~

Nails discolored from your last bold manicure? Next time don't forget the base coat, which will help prevent the color from staining your natural nails, but in the meantime, soak your nails in a small bowl filled with baking soda and warm water and use an old toothbrush or nail brush to gently scrub the discoloration away.

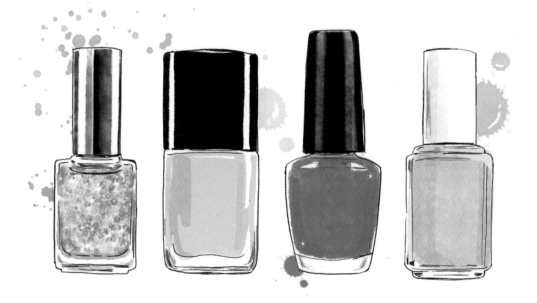

What Type of Manicure Is Right for You?

TRADITIONAL POLISH

If you're a polish-prude, you'll want to stick with traditional nail polish your first few times around the block. The same goes if you're on the opposite end of the spectrum and like to change up your lacquer regularly.

Pro:

◆ Plain old nail polish is the easiest to apply, the simplest to remove, and the healthiest for your nails.

Con:

◆ Even the best manicure on the strongest nails will only last about a week.

Tips

◆ *Skip the nail soak. Sure, it softens your cuticles so it's easier to push them back, but it also expands your nail bed and prevents the polish from adhering properly.*

◆ *Ask your manicurist to let each coat dry before applying the next for longer wear.*

GEL

If you're a manicure maven who prioritizes long-lasting over easy-to-change polish, try a gel manicure. It's better for your nails than acrylics, but still gives you the long-lasting wear.

Pros:

- It lasts about four weeks, without chipping, giving you the look of perfectly polished nails without the need for a do-over (making it ideal for before your honeymoon!).

- Each coat is cured under a UV or LED light, so when the manicure is done your nails are fully dry and you don't have to be afraid of ruining them two minutes later!

- Gel polish, like regular polish, comes in an infinite array of colors, with some of the best nail salons offering intricate art, too (think: a lace pattern to match your dress, for example!).

Cons:

- Because it lasts four weeks, your nails will show growth, with your natural nail peeking through at your cuticles little by little. The more quickly your nails grow, the more obvious it will be.

- It's expensive, with most gel manicures costing up to five times the cost of a regular manicure.

- Some places are more careful with your nails than others and, ideally, you want to find a place that only *very* minimally (if at all) buffs your nail bed (aka files the top of your nail). Even with little to no buffing, though, gel polish still prevents your nails from breathing as usual, which isn't great for them.

- The removal process can be damaging to your nails, even if you have the polish taken off by a professional.

Tip

- *To diminish the appearance of the new growth, ask for an ombré style, with a clear gel closest to your cuticle, fading into a color by your tips, or stick with a shade close to the color of your natural nail, which is more flattering, too.*

ACRYLICS

They're less expensive than gels but more damaging for your nails. I think the extra cost for gels is worth the fee, but if you're set on long-lasting polish and want to save, here's what you need to know.

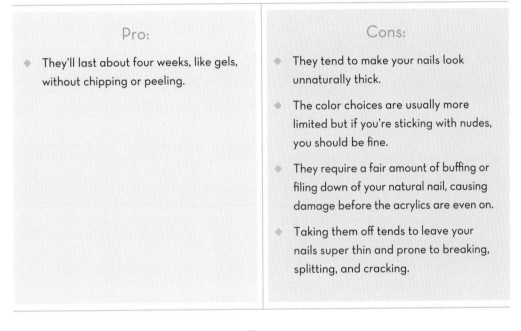

Pro:

- They'll last about four weeks, like gels, without chipping or peeling.

Cons:

- They tend to make your nails look unnaturally thick.

- The color choices are usually more limited but if you're sticking with nudes, you should be fine.

- They require a fair amount of buffing or filing down of your natural nail, causing damage before the acrylics are even on.

- Taking them off tends to leave your nails super thin and prone to breaking, splitting, and cracking.

Tips

- *Let the nail technician know that you're concerned about the damage to your nail and that you'd like your nails buffed as minimally as possible.*

- *Never pick off faux nails yourself when you're "over" them. Instead, go back to the nail salon and have them properly removed to minimize damage.*

UV OR LED GEL POLISHES

(aka CND Shellac, OPI GelColor, Essie Gel Polish)

Applied like a polish, but finishing like a gel, gel polish is what we imagine would happen if nail polish and gels had a baby.

Pros:	Con:
◆ There is no drying time.	◆ The color choices are a bit limited (but constantly expanding).
◆ It lasts up to three weeks without a chip.	
◆ There is no filing needed at all (some salons will still buff your nails for better adhesion, but feel free to ask them to skip it to save your nails).	
◆ While it is a bit pricier than a traditional polish manicure, and it does take a bit longer to apply because you cure your nails under a UV or LED light between coats, it's faster and cheaper than gels or acrylics.	

Tip

◆ *Never pick off gel polish. Unlike traditional polish, gel polish adheres far more strongly to your nail bed, causing damage if not removed properly (ideally in a salon).*

Nail Woes Troubleshooting

HANGNAILS OR CUTICLES OUT OF CONTROL?

Apply oil (coconut or olive oil from your kitchen will do the trick!) to your nails before you get into the shower and massage it in as the steam helps the oil to penetrate. Most important, resist the temptation to pull or bite! Instead, take a nail clipper and gently clip the hangnail at the root if—and only if—it is *really* needed.

NAILS SPLIT OR CRACKED?

On a clean, polish-free nail, apply a single drop of nail glue (or just Krazy Glue, available at any drugstore) on the damaged area. While it's wet, use tweezers to apply a small piece of a tissue over the nail glue. After it's dry, gently buff the glue/tissue combo with a fine nail file until smooth.

MESSED UP A NAIL?

Whether you dent your polish right after a manicure or a day later notice a chip missing, there's no need to start from scratch. Dab a tiny drop of nail polish remover across the nail to soften the remaining polish and allow it to even-out with the chip. Apply a new layer of nail color to the entire nail and let dry. Finish with top coat. If it's been more than two days, apply top coat to all nails.

WORRIED ABOUT THE UV LIGHTS AT THE NAIL SALON?

Apply SPF to your hands thirty minutes before your manicure to protect yourself.

WANT YOUR NAILS TO GROW MORE QUICKLY?

Make sure your diet is rich in both iron and calcium and ask your doctor if it would be safe for you to take a Biotin supplement, which helps encourage hair and nail growth.

NAILS SEVERELY DAMAGED?

Talk with your doctor about a prescription-strength nail polish called Genadur, which helps to prevent nails from splitting or cracking.

How to DIY a Flawless Mani

BAN THE BUFFER. Sure, buffing your nails (in moderation!) can smooth ridges, but it also strips your nails of their top layers, potentially leaving them brittle and weak.

STAY DRY. Don't soak your nails before applying polish (a common practice in nail salons). Sure, it softens your cuticles so it's easier to push them back, but it also expands your nail bed right before painting. The problem: the polish dries before your nail bed shrinks back to normal size, causing the polish to chip more easily and peel up more often. Worried about your cuticles? Push them back in the shower the night before your manicure.

GET CLEAN. Polish needs a clean, dry surface in order to adhere properly. So, before applying any polish, rub either acetone (nail polish remover) or rubbing alcohol over your nail to remove any moisture, oil, or dust.

GET GELLED. Apply petroleum jelly (aka Vaseline!) to the skin around your nail before you polish (making sure to avoid your actual nail). The nail polish won't stick to the Vaseline, making cleanup fast and easy.

LAY THE FOUNDATION. I know, you're pressed for time and skipping the base coat seems like an easy way to save time. But you'd be wrong! Skipping the base coat can cause your nails to break, your nail beds to stain, and your manicure to chip faster than ever. Plus, base coats contain important nutrients that your nails need.

TAKE IT SLOW. Apply nail polish in thin, even strokes. If the polish is too thick, it won't have a chance to adhere properly to your nail. In between coats, let each layer of polish dry.

COAT IT OVER. Once your color of choice polish is on, apply a non-quick-dry topcoat. While "quick-dry" topcoats speed evaporation on the surface, the lower layers of polish aren't drying at the same pace, saving you drying time now, but leading to more chips later.

TOP IT OFF. Every few days, apply another coat of topcoat to enhance the shine and extend the life of your mani. Here, a quick-dry formula works just as well since the nails are already dry.

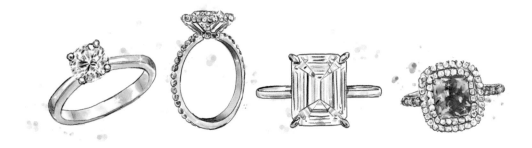

Ring TLC: How to Keep Your New Rock Sparkling

Want that new piece of ring bling to sparkle and shine for all of eternity—and especially for those ring pics you're about to share with the world in announcing your engagement? It's essential you know how to clean it! Sure, you can head to the jewelry store where your fiancé bought it for a professional cleaning (and you should, twice a year, but more on that later), but unless you happen to live or work around the corner from the jewelry store, that's horribly time-consuming! Instead, add sparkle to that stone at home, quickly, easily, and inexpensively.

FOR DAZZLING DIAMONDS

Sure, they're the hardest material on earth (they can't be scratched or broken by anything other than another diamond!), but that doesn't mean they don't need a bit of TLC to maintain their luster. Once a week, soak your diamond ring in a mixture of one part ammonia and two parts cold water for ten minutes. Rinse in cool water and let it air-dry. Ammonia can damage other stones so only use this with diamond-only engagement rings (all metals will be fine).

FOR RADIANT RUBIES, SAPPHIRES, EMERALDS, + MORE

Soak your ring in warm water and mild dishwashing liquid for five minutes before scrubbing the stone and the setting with a soft toothbrush (emphasis on *soft* since anything more abrasive can scratch softer stones). This is safe for diamonds as well, for all of you with mixed-stone rings.

WHEN IN A RUSH

Submerge your ring in a shot glass of vodka (no need to use the good stuff!) for a few minutes. Rinse it under cool water and dry it with a lint-free cloth.

TWICE A YEAR

Regardless of your ring's stone, style, metal, shape, or size, twice a year visit your jeweler to have the integrity of your ring's prongs checked to ensure your stones are secure and to avoid a dislodged diamond (a disaster if you lose it!). No longer living near the jeweler where your ring was bought? Fret not. Most large jewelry chains will happily check for a nominal fee (some even for free!).

Ring Dos + Don'ts

DO:

- remove your ring prior to applying lotions, which, even when seemingly wiped off, can leave a thin, dulling film on your stones.

- consider taking out insurance on your ring—or adding it to your homeowner's or renter's policy, if applicable—to protect yourself in the event your ring is lost or stolen. Just make sure to read the fine print since some policies don't cover all losses and others don't cover repairs.

- remove your ring when it runs the risk of being exposed to chemicals. Whether coloring your hair, using bleach, or otherwise working with harsh products, remove your ring (and put it somewhere safe!) to protect it. Some chemicals can dull diamonds and permanently damage other precious stones, like emeralds.

DON'T:

- ever take your ring off near a sink. The last thing you want to risk is a ring down the drain!

- pick your ring up by the stone. Rather, always pick up from the band to prevent the oils of your skin from dirtying the stone. This will also prevent your rock from loosening from the base.

- remove your ring in public. Whether washing your hands or showing off your sparkler, you run the risk of dropping it into a sink or a grate and make yourself more vulnerable to theft.

- compare and contrast. Every engagement ring is beautiful because of all it represents: your love, devotion, and commitment to spending your life with another. It's not a status symbol, so don't worry about what everyone else has (or doesn't have).

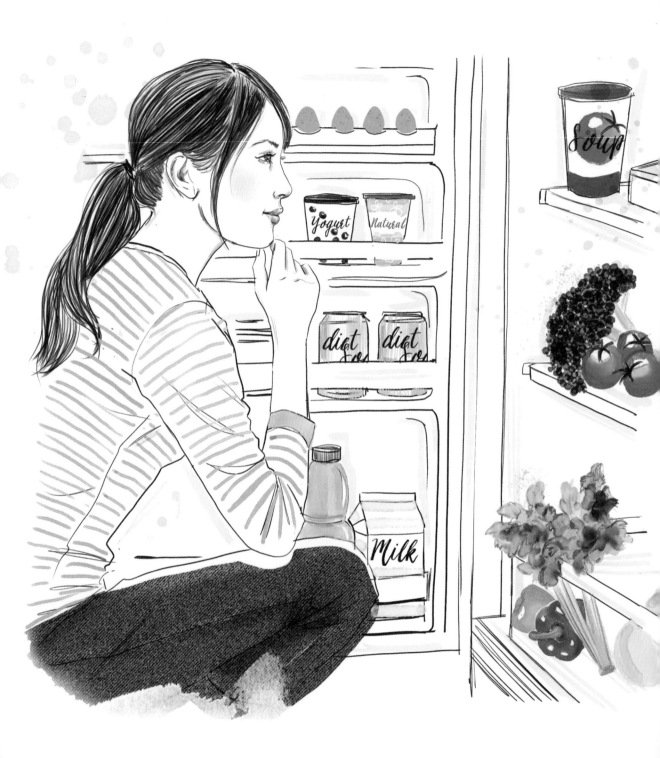

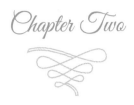

Chapter Two

SO, YOU WANT TO LOSE WEIGHT?
A 21-DAY DETOX + DIET

IT SEEMS LIKE EVERY SOON-TO-BE-BRIDE I talk to is on an "I will do anything to lose weight" diet—but it's definitely not a beauty diet! Rather, they're cutting fat and calories, and wondering why they're looking dull and drab—not to mention feeling miserable.

First of all, I want to emphasize that you're currently engaged because your main squeeze fell in love with YOU. All of you. Exactly as you are. So, before you read one more word, I want to make sure you know that you do not need to lose weight for anything or anyone. In fact, you do not need to lose weight at all. You do, though, deserve to feel amazing and that I can help you with!

Why All Other Diets Are BS and This One Will Work

———◇———

If you want to change how you eat because you want to radiate from within and feel like a million bloat-free bucks well, my dear lady, you've come to the right place.

It turns out that most of you have been thinking about your wedding diet all wrong.

Here's the deal: if there were one diet that worked for everyone, there would be one best-selling diet book and everyone would be thin and disease-free. As you know, this couldn't be further from the truth—and it's not because of a lack of willpower. Rather, it's because we're failing to account for the biodiversity among us. We're not all the same (you might be five foot four inches and your BFF five foot ten inches, you're great at math and your soon-to-be-spouse is a writing whiz, and you like avocados while they make your sister dry-heave). We're not all the same and neither are our bodies. And, no, it's not just preferences, either; it's our genetic makeup, our upbringings, and the makeup of the bacteria in our guts that help to determine why one person (ahem, my dad) can eat a pint of Häagen-Dazs ice cream every night, feel awesome afterward, and complain about losing weight the next morning, and another (ahem, me) feels wretched after a single bite of ice cream and bloated for days after. Or why two people can have the exact same diets and exercise plans and still be two very different sizes.

The secret no one else is telling you: it's not about how many calories you're consuming or whether or not you're eating too many fats. And it's most definitely not about willpower. It's about inflammation, your gut's immune response, and figuring out what foods your body thrives on by immediately putting them to use as energy and what foods your body fights (and turns into bloated bellies).

That's why calorie or fat-restricting diets often don't work and, if they do, their results are temporary and you end up gaining it all back—or more!

So instead of trying to sell you a one-size-fits-all "diet" that will only work for some of you (like many diet books!), I'm here to tell you that there is no such thing as one diet that works for every-one—no matter what those best-selling diet books claim.

No, that doesn't mean you need to spend the next years upon years testing all the diets out there to find the one for you through a time-consuming and morale-busting process of elimination. Rather, I'm going to give you the tools nutritionists use (without your having to spend your precious time or money on one-on-one professional sessions). Hey, there's a reason *People* magazine called me the "DIY Beauty Queen"—I like to DIY it, and give others the tools needed to DIY it, too!

In just twenty-one days, I'm going to help you detox and reboot.

I'm going to show you how to lose weight (if you need to), feel amazing, and look *RADIANT*.

Your skin will glow. You'll stop feeling bloated. You'll look incredible.

And through this detox, you'll discover your ideal long-term diet for sustained radiance ever after.

The secret: figuring out the foods (from a slew of common allergens) your body is negatively responding to, causing you to break out, your skin to look dull, your belly to bloat, and more, and elim-inating them while indulging in all the other foods your body loves whenever and however you want.

With this plan, you will look and feel like the best version of *you*. You will be exactly the right size for your body. You will be radiant.

Sure, the first three weeks are going to be challenging—and they'll likely rock your world (in the best way possible). But it's only three weeks, and you can do *anything* for just three weeks.

Why three weeks? For two reasons: first, it takes twenty-one days to eliminate built-up toxins in your body, reboot your system, and see the effects of a dietary change on your body and beauty. Second, it also takes twenty-one days to form a new habit, so a commitment to any long-lasting change needs to begin with a commitment to twenty-one days, after which sticking with it becomes second nature.

So, get out your calendar and block off the next three weeks because you're about to get to know your body in an epic new way. For the best results, do this detox at least five months before your wedding, but the sooner the better!

The Radiant Bride Detox +
What to Eat . . . and Not Eat

So, what exactly are you eating (or not eating)?

Simply put, you're cutting out the most common allergens and bowel bloaters that are often responsible for your body holding on to excess weight and keeping track of how we feel to determine *your* best diet to get you into your best body.

This will be a largely gluten-free, dairy-free diet. You're going to avoid soy, eggs, processed sugar, peanuts, some meats, nightshade vegetables, and a few fruits. But only for twenty-one days. This is all just temporary since we need to cut out all the potential allergens in your body and then gradually reintroduce them in order to figure out your weight-hoarding triggers.

Sure, this list can be a bit overwhelming at first, but take some time to get familiar with it, clean out your kitchen of the "don'ts" and load up on the "dos," and get ready to whip that body of yours into its best shape ever.

So, what are you eating?!

Lots! You're going to load up on anti-inflammatory vegetables, healthy (and belly-filling) fats, and lean proteins. You're not going to count calories (not a single one!) or consider portion size. You're going to eat anything you want from the "dos" column in unlimited quantities, whenever you want.

And don't worry, you're not banning these foods forever! I'll show you how to reintroduce them, pronto in the Radiant Bride Diet (see page 42).

Wondering why you can't just get allergy testing done at the doctor's office and go from there? Because it's not only expensive but also highly unreliable and an elimination diet is actually the gold standard for figuring out the best diet for you.

Dieting for your wedding day shouldn't leave you obsessing over grams of fat or counting calories. And it shouldn't make you grumpy or miserable. It also shouldn't have you crash-dieting and obsessively weighing yourself. Instead, this Radiant Bride Detox + Diet is all about finding the foods that are causing you to feel bloated, your skin to look less than luminous, and your body to hold on to weight it doesn't need.

	EAT	DON'T EAT
Vegetables	Raw, steamed, juiced, sautéed, or roasted vegetables (especially green leafy ones), sea vegetables (like dulse, kelp, and nori), sweet potatoes, yams, fresh and dried herbs	Nightshade vegetables (tomatoes, eggplant, peppers)
Fruit	Fresh or frozen whole fruits and berries, avocados, olives	Citrus fruit (oranges, grapefruits), fruit juice, grapes
Grains + Starches	Gluten-free grains, including rice, quinoa, millet, amaranth, teff, buckwheat	White rice, wheat, corn, barley, spelt, Kamut, rye, oats, potatoes
Meat, Fish, + Poultry	Cold water fish (fresh or water-packed, including salmon, tuna, trout, halibut, sardines, mackerel, pike, kippers)	Pork, beef, veal, sausage, cold cuts, canned meat, sausage or hot dogs, shellfish, eggs
Dairy	Nut milks (like almond, cashew, etc.), hemp milk, rice milk, coconut milk	Milk (from animals), cheese, yogurt, butter, ice cream, nondairy creamers

	EAT	DON'T EAT
Vegetable Protein, Legumes, Nuts, + Seeds	Nuts, seeds, nut butters, seed butters, lentils, beans, split peas, spirulina, blue-green algae, bee pollen	Peanuts, peanut butter, soy (including soy sauce, tofu, tempeh, soybean oil)
Sweeteners + Condiments	100 percent pure stevia, coconut nectar, 100 percent dried, non-citrus fruit, sea salt, any fresh or dried herbs	White sugar, brown sugar, brown rice syrup, evaporated cane juice, maple syrup, honey, agave, fructose, molasses, corn syrup, artificial sweeteners (like Splenda, Equal), juice concentrate, ketchup, processed seasonings
Fats + Oils	Avocados, nuts, seeds, olives, cold-pressed oils (including olive, coconut, flax, sesame, safflower, sunflower, walnut, almond)	Butter, margarine, ghee, shortening, canola oil, processed oils, packaged salad dressing, mayonnaise, packaged roasted nuts and seeds
Drinks	Water, green tea, herbal tea, white tea, green juice, yerba mate	Coffee, black tea, alcohol, soda, carbonated beverages, fruit juice

PREP

Before you start the twenty-one-day Radiant Bride Detox you need to prepare mentally, physically, and logistically. Before you get started, it's important to . . .

THROW AWAY YOUR SCALE. I know you want to lose weight, but trust me on this. When you're stressed out over the number on the scale, your body doesn't know the difference between the stress it feels from feeling fat and the stress your ancestors used to feel during a slow hunting season, when holding on to fat was evolutionarily adaptive for survival. As a result, your cortisol levels spike and your body goes into immediate fight or flight mode. And when those cortisol levels spike, losing weight is all but impossible. Plus, the number on the scale tells you nothing about how f'ing hot you look, so let's start by throwing that sucker away and instead measuring our health, wellness, and beauty by how we feel.

PREPARE YOURSELF MENTALLY. What we're about to do is going to be challenging, but it's only for a very short period of time and, after that, you will know exactly how to eat for beauty and health. Twenty-one days is nothing to "pay" for that, right?!

BUY A JOURNAL. The most important part about this detox is figuring out what works for you, and to do so, you're going to need to keep track. It's essential that you're able to keep this with you all the time, so make sure that it's small and handy. You can even use the "notes" on your phone, if that's easier for you—just be sure it's set to back up so you don't risk losing it.

TELL FRIENDS AND FAMILY. While this detox in no way needs to put your social life on hold, it does require you to take some extra steps to ensure you know what you're eating in order to accurately document how your body responds. Rather than having to explain at each social occasion why you're passing on the booze, fill in your nearest and dearest and ask for their help and support. Or, better yet, get them on board, too! You definitely don't need to be getting married to do this detox!

ALTER PLANS, IF NEEDED. Look at your calendar for the next three weeks. Planning a dinner with your BFFs at your favorite Mexican restaurant? Ask them to come over for dinner instead so you know what you're eating (restaurants often add gluten or dairy unknowingly) or call the restaurant ahead of time to discuss the menu options that will be best for you.

CLEAN OUT YOUR KITCHEN. Having to rely on willpower sucks. Give yourself the greatest odds of success by doing a major clean out. If you live with your fiancé, family members, or roommates, you're going to have to get them on board, too (or just ask them to keep their special stash in hiding), so you're not tempted. While you're at it, check out any supplements you usually take to ensure they're gluten- and dairy-free as well.

KNOW YOU MAY FEEL WORSE BEFORE YOU FEEL BETTER. Many of us are walking around with pounds of toxins in our bodies (some experts say an average of five to twenty pounds!). It's completely normal to feel like crap as your body works to eliminate them. It's also normal to gain weight as your body releases built-up toxins until you're able to eliminate them. This is a normal—and temporary!—part of the process.

STEP 2

CLEAN OUT

Spend time getting familiar with the chart on pages 34-35 and clean out your kitchen of everything labeled "Don't Eat" and load up on everything in the "Eat" list—having lots of delicious healthy options easily accessible will make sticking with this plan exponentially easier.

DETOX

For the next twenty-one days eat *ANYTHING* you want from the "Eat" list, without worrying about portion control (whatever that means!), fat, calories, or anything else you've worried about before. Be creative, try new recipes (pick up my first book, *The Recipe for Radiance*, for lots of beauty-boosting recipes!), and crowd out all the foods you own on your "Don't Eat" list with loads of delicious new ones. Experiment with herbs to deliciously and detox-friendly flavor foods. And remember, if you can't pronounce it or can't recognize it, skip it. Unlike other diets, this detox is about tapping into your body and your needs. Prefer to graze throughout the day? Go for it! Rather have three sit-down meals? Wonderful! Like to play it by ear based on how you're feeling? Even better, since hormonal fluctuations, activity levels, and stress all affect how much food we need.

DRINK LOTS OF WATER. It not only helps your skin to radiate, it also helps to support your body's detoxifying mechanisms. Aim to drink at least eight 8-ounce cups a day.

PAY ATTENTION TO HOW YOU FEEL . . . AND WRITE IT DOWN! Unlike food journals you've perhaps done in the past, this isn't about keeping track of what you eat in order to stay within a restricted calorie or point allotment so much as it is about keeping track of how you feel when you eat certain foods. The goal in embarking on an elimination diet is to see what works for you and what doesn't and the best way to spot patterns is to write it all down so you can go back later and evaluate what you've found. The key here is to write down both what you eat and how you feel both immediately after eating anything as well as if how you feel changes later. Ask yourself these questions when you're journaling:

How does my stomach feel?   What are my cravings?

How are my energy levels?   How am I sleeping?

How is my skin?   What's my mood?

Have I been going to the bathroom regularly?   Do I feel clear and sharp?

LET YOUR BODY REST AND HEAL. It takes your body eight hours to fully digest food. Give yourself a full twelve hours between dinner at night and breakfast the next morning to allow your body to fully process and release toxins.

MAKE SURE YOU GO TO THE BATHROOM. Going to the bathroom is an essential part of detoxing but any change in a diet plan can cause your bowels to either go into overdrive or stop altogether. This is largely based on how you've been eating before now. If you're constipated, make sure you're drinking enough water, eating enough fiber (leafy greens, dried fruit), and exercising (even just brisk walking). If you're still not going, pick up some Natural Calm at the health food store and use as directed.

EAT CALMLY. When you're constantly eating on the run or while judging your food choices, you're putting your body into stress mode and sending a message to it to hold on to every last bit of body mass. Sit down, enjoy it, savor it. You'll reduce your body's stress response and allow your body to focus on digestion (and enjoyment!).

CHEW. Just like you can exfoliate your skin to break down dead and dull skin cells chemically (with fruit acids, for example) and manually (with anything granular), your food is also best digested when both manually and chemically broken down. When you swallow your food without chewing it thoroughly, you skip the mechanical breakdown and rely solely on the chemical processes that take place in your stomach, putting undue strain on your belly. The result: bloat, constipation, diarrhea, and more! The goal should be to chew your food until liquefied in your mouth (gross as it sounds) to help your body to more efficiently use the energy you need and eliminate the rest.

TAKE A PROBIOTIC. Talk with your doctor about adding a probiotic to your daily routine. For many of us (especially if you've taken antibiotics in the past, have eaten a lot of meat and dairy, or just have persistent stomach issues) our gut bacteria is out of balance and a single pill a day can help put everything back in balance.

EASE INTO IT, IF NEEDED. If your diet up until this point has been largely fast-food and processed, packaged snacks, take an additional week before starting the cleanse to slowly cut back on processed foods and add in healthier foods.

EASE OFF OF CAFFEINE. If you're struggling with caffeine dependency and feeling the effects of stopping cold turkey, gradually switch from coffee to caffeinated tea or yerba mate to help ease the transition. Alternatively, try starting your morning with spicy warm water with lemon (just add a dash of cayenne to a mug full of hot water and lemon juice) or an energy-packed chocolate "milk" by stirring a tablespoon of raw cacao powder into a mug of hot almond milk.

WHAT YOUR CRAVINGS ARE TELLING YOU

If you're craving sweets: *you probably need more sleep and emotional support. When all you want to do is dive into a bag of candy, it's usually your body looking for a quick energy boost or the food equivalent of a hug from sugar's immediate endorphin boost. Try getting more z's and get a real hug from your significant other instead! No time to sleep or no one to hug right away? Fresh fruit and sweet vegetables (like sweet potatoes and carrots) can often satiate a sweet tooth, healthfully.*

If you're craving chocolate: *you may need more magnesium, which can be found in nuts, seeds, and legumes.*

If you're craving carbs: *you're probably not getting enough protein and/or are just feeling down. Next time you're craving a big bowl of pasta, get your serotonin and dopamine boost by getting a massage, taking a bath, or catching up with a girlfriend, all with a protein-packed snack.*

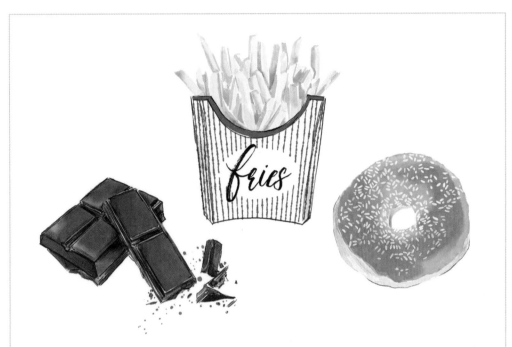

If you're craving greasy, fatty foods: *you're likely in need of more calcium and fat. Find calcium in sesame seeds, almonds, Brazil nuts, sunflower seeds, kale, watercress, broccoli, and dried figs. And remember that not all fats are created equal, so load up on healthy fat from avocados, nuts, and seeds.*

If you're craving coffee: *you're likely drained and dehydrated. Drink more water to rehydrate you and take a break from whatever it is you're doing and you'll feel better, stat!*

If you're craving something salty: *you may need some chlorine in your diet, which is found in kelp, celery, and fish.*

EVALUATE

When the twenty-one days are over, look through your journal (you can do this throughout the cleanse, too, if you'd like) and pay attention to any patterns that may emerge. Notice that every time you eat brown rice you want to crawl into bed? You are likely sensitive to grains, even gluten-free ones, or have a rice allergy. Feel great all day when you eat gluten-free granola and almond milk for breakfast (whereas your former cereal and cow's milk breakfast left you drained and counting down the minutes until lunch)? You're likely gluten or dairy intolerant. Or both!

While the Radiant Bride Detox eliminates all the most common allergens and inflammatory foods and the vast majority of you will feel fabulous on this plan, every body is different and it is, of course, possible to have an adverse reaction to a typically non-inflammatory food on the Eat list. If you notice anything on the cleanse diet that made you feel less than awesome, cut it out. Otherwise, you're likely already feeling better than ever!

If you're feeling like a million bucks—or at least on the path toward your millionaire status—and your wedding is less than two months away, try to stick with your eating plan on the Radiant Bride Detox and come back to step five after your honeymoon!

The Radiant Bride Diet

PART 1:

PARTIAL REINTRODUCTION

As promised, you don't need to avoid the "Don't Eat" foods forever—although you'll want to continue to avoid dairy, gluten, and processed sugar as much as possible, if not altogether, until you're back from your honeymoon. And keep caffeine and alcohol to a minimum, too, until after the big day.

Before you dig into a giant bowl of peanuts, though, it's essential that you know how to reintroduce these foods back into your diet in a way that not only won't reverse all the progress we've already made, but also ensures you continue on the path to looking and feeling your best for your big day.

The key is reintroducing each food group intentionally, individually, and thoughtfully so you can easily identify your personal triggers. For the next four days you will reintroduce one food at a time and pay close attention to how your body responds. That body of yours is pretty incredible at telling you what works and what doesn't—you just need to listen!

To start, pick one food from the list of foods to reintroduce first (for example, eggs) and start with that. Let's call this "NF" (for, "New Food"—clever, I know).

Foods to Reintroduce First

- NIGHTSHADE VEGETABLES (tomatoes, eggplant, peppers)
- CITRUS FRUIT (oranges, grapefruits)
- POTATOES

- PORK
- BEEF
- VEAL
- SHELLFISH
- EGGS

- PEANUTS + PEANUT BUTTER
- SOY (including soy sauce, tofu, tempeh, soybean oil)
- GRAPES

For the next two days, add your chosen NF in at least two meals each day, journaling regularly. Then go back to your cleanse diet for two days, continuing to evaluate regularly since it can take a day or two for a reaction to show up.

Day 1:	Add NF back in at least two meals, journal regularly
Day 2:	Add NF back in at least two meals, journal regularly
Day 3:	Cleanse diet + Evaluate
Day 4:	Cleanse diet + Evaluate

Each day, journal your answer to these questions:

How do you feel while you're eating?

How do you feel immediately after?

How are your energy levels now, in an hour, in three hours, in six hours?

How did you sleep?

Did you go to the bathroom?

How do you feel in general?

On day four, decide whether or not to continue eating this particular NF based on your journal entries, not based on your emotional attachment or memories of the food.

If you decide to add it back into your diet because you feel well, it now becomes part of your *personalized* Radiant Bride Diet.

Repeat with another NF for the next four days until you've reintroduced all the foods you care to reintroduce.

If you notice a negative reaction to one of the NF categories, you can repeat with each individual component. For example, if you test nightshade vegetables and feel bloated, next you can try reintroducing just eggplant and see how that goes on its own.

For mildly negative reactions (like feeling a bit tired, for example), experiment with adding the food in moderation (only having it once a week, for example) and see how you respond then.

The goal here is to find out the best foods for you, that let any excess weight drop off naturally and seamlessly—and all without ever feeling like you're depriving yourself. In reintroducing these common inflammatory foods and weight-loss hinderers—and paying close attention to how we feel—you're going to discover your personalized diet for radiance.

Note: Heading off on your bachelorette weekend? Stick to your plan as much as possible and forgive yourself of any "mistakes"—happiness makes everyone pretty so do what makes you happy and restart the cleanse when you return.

PART 2:

AFTER THE BIG DAY . . . AND THE HONEYMOON

When you look and feel as good as you do now, you're likely going to want to stick with your current gluten-free, dairy-free eating plan, making this last step entirely optional. For the rest of you, now's the time to gently reintroduce the rest of these foods into your Radiant Bride Diet and to see how you feel.

Just because your wedding is over though, doesn't mean it's time to throw caution to the wind and dig into a grilled cheese sandwich. Rather, reintroduce these remaining foods the same way as in step 5 to ensure your hard work isn't lost.

Foods to Reintroduce Post-Honeymoon (optional)

◆ GLUTEN-CONTAINING GRAINS: wheat, corn, barley, spelt, Kamut, rye, oats

◆ DAIRY: cow's milk, cheese, yogurt, butter, ice cream, nondairy creamers

◆ SWEETENERS: maple syrup, honey, brown rice syrup

◆ FATS/OILS: butter, margarine, ghee, mayonnaise

◆ DRINKS: Coffee, alcohol (in moderation)

Foods to Consider Continuing to Avoid

◆ GLUTEN-CONTAINING GRAINS: White rice, white flour

◆ PROCESSED MEATS: sausage, cold cuts, canned meat, hot dogs

◆ SWEETENERS: white sugar, brown sugar, evaporate cane juice, fructose, molasses, corn syrup, artificial sweeteners (like Splenda, Equal), juice concentrate.

◆ FATS/OILS: shortening, canola oil, processed oils, packaged salad dressing

◆ DRINKS: soda, carbonated beverages, fruit juice

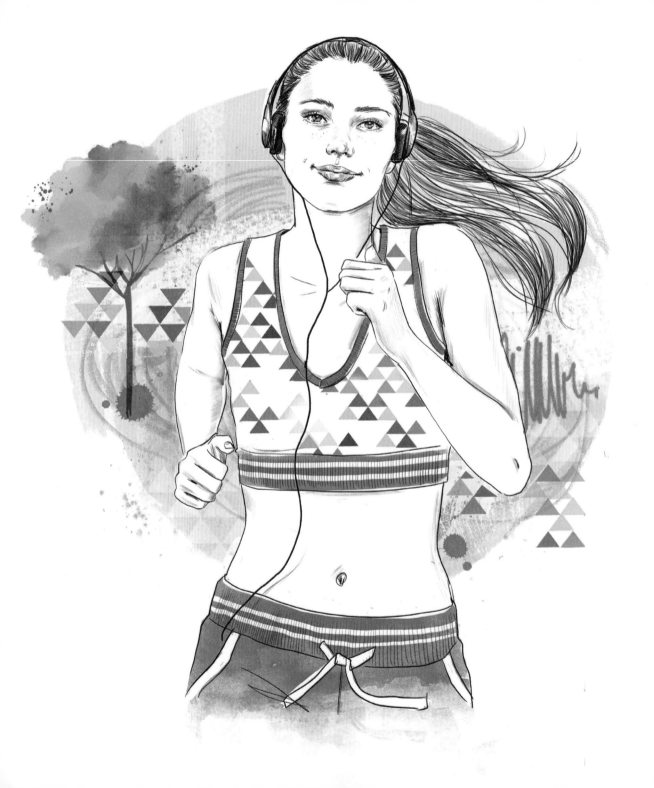

Chapter Three

THE BUFF BRIDE FITNESS PLAN

YOU DON'T NEED ME TO TELL YOU that with a full-time fitness trainer and unlimited time and funds you could easily have buns of steel and guns the NRA would be jealous of. But the fact is that most of us not only don't have the ability to focus so intently on looking fit, we also don't want to, which is not to say that you don't want to show off toned arms in that strapless dress of yours or a firm derrière in that mermaid gown.

The key: getting the biggest bang for your buck (and time!)—and I have all the insider secrets from my years of working as a beauty expert and the countless hours I've spent working and pallin' around with celebrity fitness trainers.

The secret to the Buff Bride Fitness Plan: quick and easy workouts that are not only designed to be done on a busy bride's schedule, but are also tailored to your dress in order to ensure the parts of your body that are on full display get all the pre-wedding love they deserve. But going into this, I must remind you that *being* healthy is way more important than *looking* healthy, and the two do not always coexist.

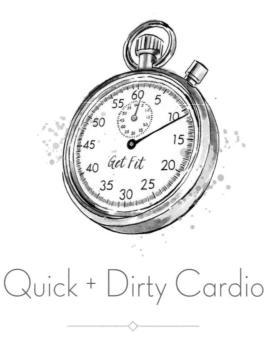

Quick + Dirty Cardio

Add cardiovascular workouts to your wedding-prep routine to keep that love-filled heart of yours in tip-top shape. But on a how-to-look-show-stoppingly-stunning-on-your-wedding-day note, cardio also helps you to flush away toxins (and, thus, excess weight, too), by boosting your metabolism and promoting detoxification.

That said, you don't need to be spending hours in the gym or training for a marathon in order to reap all the benefits. To get the biggest bang for your bridal buck, HIIT (aka high-intensity interval training) is about to be your new BFF! Combining intense bursts of all-out exertion followed by resting recovery, HIIT can get you in the best shape of your life in just twenty minutes, three days per week.

So how do you do HIIT exactly? Well, there aren't any real rules to HIIT other than that after a brief warm-up, you do high-intensity intervals where you push yourself as hard as you can, recover, and then repeat. The best part about HIIT is that you never outgrow the workout since you can always increase your speed, incline, and/or resistance to make the workout harder. And you can take this workout anywhere. From the treadmill to the StairMaster, the rowing machine to the pool, the track to the bike!

Ready to get started?

HIIT: BEGINNER

If you're new to exercising, this is a great place to start. Remember that the times you're asked to push yourself can be anything from a brisk walk, perhaps at an incline, to a full-on sprint. It's all about what's hard for you.

0:00–5:00	Warm up at a slow and steady pace.
5:00–5:30	Push yourself as hard and fast as you safely can.
5:30–6:30	Catch your breath either by stopping entirely or dramatically reducing your level of exertion.
6:30–17:00	Repeat minutes 5:00 to 6:30 seven more times.
17:00–20:00	Cool down.

HIIT: INTERMEDIATE

If you're a regular exerciser but are looking to take your fitness to a whole new level, start here!

0:00–5:00	Warm up at a slow and steady pace.
5:00–6:00	Push yourself as hard and fast as you safely can.
6:00–7:00	Catch your breath either by stopping entirely or dramatically reducing your level of exertion.
7:00–17:00	Repeat minutes 5:00 to 7:00 five more times.
17:00–20:00	Cool down.

HITT: INTERMEDIATE PLUS

If you're already a fitness fan, this is for you.

0:00–3:00	Warm up at a slow and steady pace.
3:00–4:30	Push yourself as hard and fast as you safely can.
4:30–5:30	Catch your breath either by stopping entirely or dramatically reducing your level of exertion.
5:30–18:00	Repeat minutes 3:00 to 5:30 five more times.
18:00–20:00	Cool down.

HITT: ADVANCED

Know everyone at your gym—and their entire life stories? You may be ready for this!

0:00–2:00	Warm up at a slow and steady pace.
2:00–4:00	Push yourself as hard and fast as you safely can.
4:00–4:30	Catch your breath either by stopping entirely or dramatically reducing your level of exertion.
4:30–17:00	Repeat minutes 2:00 to 4:30 five more times.
17:00–20:00	Cool down.

Remember, you can always increase your speed, incline, or resistance within any of these plans to make them more (or less) challenging. So, feel free to experiment with the length of these intervals and mix it up by switching between the StairMaster and bike or adding an incline to a treadmill.

Hate working out? Find some kids to play tag with! It's HIIT at its finest (and fittest)!

Timed Toning

Just as your cardio routine doesn't need to take up eons of your already spread-too-thin time, neither does your weight training. In fact, I'm about to give you a buff bridal boot camp routine that will get you in tip-top shape in just fifteen minutes a day, four days each week, and just six weeks to see results. Here's what you'll need:

◆ Light weights (2 to 5 pounds) ◆ Empty floor space ◆ Yoga mat, optional

For fifteen minutes, four times a week, you'll do four exercises from the below list. Focus on the exercises most relevant for your dress style, but feel free to do them all, if for no other reason than to boost your metabolism.

Do one exercise for sixty seconds, rest for fifteen seconds, do the second for sixty seconds, rest for fifteen seconds, and so on. Repeat three times, trying to increase the number of repetitions you're able to do in sixty seconds or the level of difficulty. Try not to repeat the same exercises two days in a row.

0:00–1:00	Exercise 1
1:00–1:15	Rest
1:15–2:15	Exercise 2
2:15–2:30	Rest
2:30–3:30	Exercise 3
3:30–3:45	Rest
3:45–4:45	Exercise 4
4:45–5:00	Rest
5:00–15:00	Repeat 0:00–5:00 two more times.

IF YOUR DRESS IS SLEEVELESS . . .

Your arms will be on full display. The key, though, is to tone and tighten, not to bulk, which is why you should stick with light weights (think 2 to 5 pounds each), or just use your own body weight, and do lots of repetitions. I recommend the following key exercises for you.

Tricep Dips

Sit on the edge of a sturdy chair with your hands on the edge of the seat, fingers tucked underneath. Walk your feet out until your backside is off the chair and your knees are bent at a ninety-degree angle, with your feet flat on the floor. Bend your elbows, lowering your body toward the floor before straightening your arms and pushing yourself back up. To make it harder, walk your feet out so they're straight in front of you.

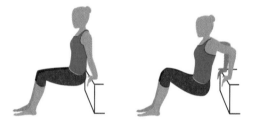

Bicep Curls

Stand with your arms at your sides with a weight in each hand, palms facing forward. Bend your elbows to raise the weights to your shoulders before lowering. To make it harder, increase the weight and repetitions.

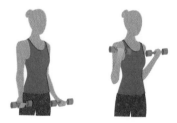

Push-Ups

Begin in a plank position, with your hands under your shoulders, but slightly wider than shoulder-width apart. Keep your back straight, your core and glutes engaged, and your toes firmly planted. Lower your body, in a straight line, until your chest gets as close as possible to the ground without touching. Be sure to keep your back and hips straight throughout the whole move. Try to keep your elbows pointing slightly backward. Pause at the bottom before pushing back up to the starting position. If this is too difficult, drop to your knees or elevate your hands on a bench.

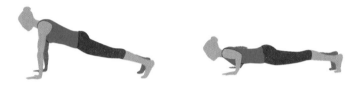

IF YOU'RE GOING STRAPLESS . . .

You'll want to focus not only on your arms, but also your shoulders, upper back, and chest. While a good tailor will ensure your dress is fitted enough to stay up without digging in and showcasing armpit fat or an upper back roll (even when it's only skin), strong muscle tone is a must.

Lateral Raise

Start standing with your feet together and arms at your sides, palms facing your legs. With a weight in each hand, raise your arms directly out to the sides, then lower them.

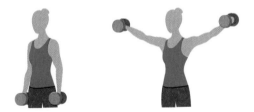

Super-woman

Lie on your stomach with your arms extended in front of you. Lift your arms, chest, and legs up a few inches, hold for three seconds, then release. To make it harder, hold light weights in each hand.

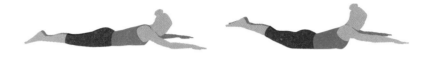

Row

Standing with feet hip-width apart and your knees slightly bent, pitch your torso forward at a forty-five-degree angle. With a weight in each hand (dangling toward the floor), bend your elbows and pinch your upper back to drag your arms against your body (so your elbows point toward the ceiling).

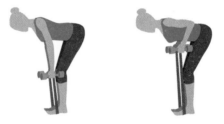

IF YOUR GOWN IS FITTED THROUGH YOUR TORSO . . .

We want to chisel and whittle, not add bulk, which is why we're skipping the traditional sit-ups (that can sometimes just add a layer of muscle on top of whatever you have) in favor of these tummy toners.

Twisting Planks

Starting at the top of a push-up position (arms straight and under your shoulders with your legs and core straight behind you), hold your core steady as you bring your right knee toward the out-side of your right elbow and then back behind you, returning to a plank position. Repeat with your left knee, bringing it toward the outside of your left elbow and back. Then bring your right knee under your body and across to the inside of your left elbow, squeezing through your core before repeating with your left knee and right elbow. Repeat the entire sequence.

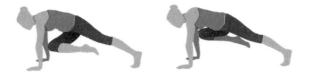

Weighted Rope Climbers

In a sit-up position, hold 1- to 3-pound weights in each hand and mimic climbing a rope between your knees. Keep your shoulder blades off the floor (or as close to off the floor as possible) as you alternate "climbing" your hands one in front of the other.

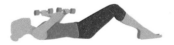

Mountain Climbers

Begin with your body in a push-up position. Step one leg in between your hands, with a bent knee, while keeping the other leg back. Hold your abs in tight and switch legs at a fast pace, keeping your hands on the floor the whole time. If this is too difficult, lift your bottom up so you're in a position somewhere between a push-up and downward dog.

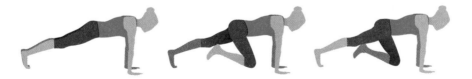

IF YOUR DRESS IS CURVE-HUGGING . . .

It's all about lifting and rounding the butt and toning the thighs.

Squats

Stand with your feet shoulder-width apart, your stomach engaged and your weight on your heels. Sit back and down, as if you were going to sit in a chair. Aim to get your thighs parallel to the floor while keeping your knees over (not in front of) your ankles. Keep your chest up and your gaze forward. Stand back up. Hold weights in your hands to make it more challenging or jump up instead of standing back up.

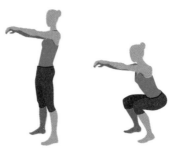

Forward + Reverse Lunges

Standing with your feet hip-width apart, step your right foot forward into a deep lunge and slowly lower your body until your front knee is bent ninety degrees (your back knee will bend, too). Pause before stepping back to the starting position. Do the same with your left leg. Repeat in reverse, stepping one foot back into the lunge and then stepping back up and repeating. Hold weights to make it more challenging.

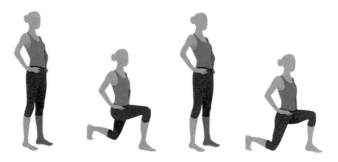

Curtsy Lunges

Stand with your feet hip-width apart before stepping your right foot back toward the left corner of the room. With your chest up and core tight and engaged, lower your body down to a lunge. Pause before returning to the starting position. Hold weights to make it more challenging.

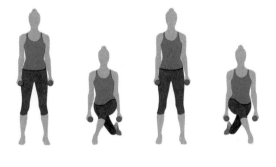

Need Help Getting Motivated?

Over 40 percent of women say that the reason they aren't as fit and healthy as they would like is because of a lack of motivation. Another 40 percent say it's because of laziness. So, how do you beat both laziness and a lack of motivation? Keep on reading! Here are ten ways to get motivated and push your laziness aside.

GET CLEAR

Ask yourself why you want to get fit. Having a clear reason for working out and getting healthy—one that matters to you!—is the best way to get motivated and stay that way. So, figure out your reason (it will be different for everyone but try to think past looking great in your wedding dress!). Maybe you want to be healthy to live a long life for your children or perhaps you want to be able to climb the stairs without getting winded at work. So, spend time figuring out why you want to get fit and remind yourself of your reason regularly.

SCHEDULE IT

Like you would a doctor appointment, put your workouts in your calendar. In pen!

HAVE FUN

Finding a workout you enjoy is one of the easiest ways to ensure you stay motivated (and not bored!). It's hard to stay motivated to do something you hate, but if you can find an exercise you love, it will be easy! Not into running in circles around a track or elliptical training? Think outside the box! Plan a dance party with friends, take an intenSati class, or make a deal with yourself that you can only watch your favorite TV show while moving!

BE YOUR OWN DJ

Download some new tunes and have fun with it. Studies have shown that listening to music while working out keeps your energy up, resulting in higher-intensity and longer-lasting workouts. So get grooving (and moving)!

SET REALISTIC GOALS

It's easy to lose motivation when your goals are so lofty that you feel defeated before you've even begun. One easy way to ensure your workout goals are manageable is to try to increase your fitness by just 10 percent each week, by either adding 10 percent more time to your workouts, 10 percent more weight while strength-training, or 10 percent more repetitions every seven days.

REWARD YOURSELF

Each of us are motivated by different things—for some of us, working toward a new pair of shoes will do the trick while others may be more motivated by the dream of a vacation. Give yourself a point for each goal you achieve (maybe you keep track of the number of miles you run or the number of dance classes you attend) and, when you hit a certain number of points, splurge on something that makes you happy! Need more constant reinforcement? Set smaller goals and reward yourself more often with smaller, more manageable rewards (like a dinner out!).

REEVALUATE OFTEN

If you're starting to feel lazy, be honest with yourself (without passing judgment) and start from scratch. Reevaluate why you want to get fit and redefine your answer. Find a new workout to try, alter your goals, or change your reward system.

DRESS UP

Hitting the gym in a ratty old T-shirt? No wonder you feel blah. Ditch the sweat-stained T-shirt and buy yourself a few cute workout outfits. When you look good, you feel good. And when you feel good, your energy is up and your workout is far better.

PLAY TOURIST

It's easy to feel like you're running in circles when you're, well, literally running in circles around a track. If you take your workouts outdoors, switch up your route and tour your city as if you were in a foreign place by exploring a new neighborhood or finding a new scenic trail.

FIND FITNESS FRIENDS

Ask your friends to meet you for a run or to come over and try to learn a new dance routine (hit up YouTube for that!). Everything is more fun with friends and exercising is no exception.

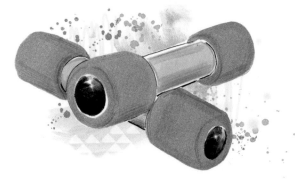

Buff Bride Bonus Detox

———◇———

If your body is working at full throttle to detox your body of years of poor food choices, you may not have many reserves left in store to fuel your workouts and to help your body to build muscle. Boost your body's detoxification mechanisms and jump-start your fitness goals by supporting the natural cleansing systems you were born with (but likely haven't been giving the TLC they need).

BREATHE

Sounds too easy to actually work? Think again! Our breath is one of our body's primary detoxifying mechanisms, helping us to literally breathe out the bad. Take deep, long breaths in, followed by deeper, longer exhales to get rid of all the stale breath.

JUMP

Your lymphatic system is commonly called "the garbage disposal of the body," churning out all the toxins and trash. To work properly, though, it needs your help to keep things moving. While any type of movement helps to turn on this internal garbage disposal, jumping is one of the best ways to throw your lymphatic system into overdrive. Just a few minutes of jumping rope or on a trampoline (or rebounder) stimulates the bowels, promotes detoxification, and helps reduce the appearance of cellulite. Not into jumping? A massage promotes lymphatic drainage, too.

SWEAT

Exercise, hit up the sauna, have some sexy time . . . whatever works for you! Your skin is one of your body's best detoxifying mechanisms and sweat is its means of purging the toxins. Shower immediately after to wash them all away.

BRUSH

Dry skin-brushing not only exfoliates your dry, dead skin cells (the ones that are blocking the pores your body uses to detox through when you sweat), it also stimulates the lymphatic system. Use a natural bristle brush and, standing in the shower, gently scrub your skin using gentle, circular, upward motions followed by longer, smoother ones. Start at the ankles and work your way up the front of your body, brushing toward your heart. On your back, start at your neck and work your way down. Shower afterward to wash away the loosened cells.

BATHE

Once a week, add two cups of Epsom salt to a warm bath and soak for twenty to thirty minutes. The salts help to pull retained fluids and toxins from your body while you blissfully relax.

DRINK FILTERED WATER

Filtered water is like gasoline for your body's internal garbage disposal. Drink at least half of your body weight in ounces of water to keep your body's detoxification mechanisms working at their max and to help flush out any toxins released by these other detoxification mechanisms.

COLON HYDRO THERAPY

They're not for the faint of heart, but for women who suffer from persistent constipation or whose weddings are mere weeks away and they're looking to take their detox to a whole other level, ask your doctor or holistic wellness practitioner to recommend a colon hydrotherapy center. There, highly trained and modest practitioners will insert a tube up your anus (you barely feel it) and slowly flush water into your rectum to help dislodge stuck fecal matter. Again, not for the faint of heart!

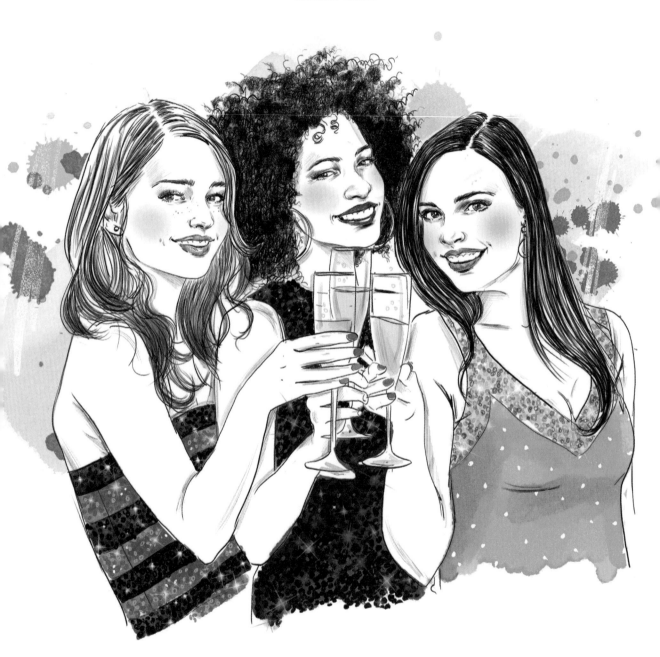

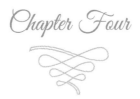

Chapter Four

BE A BEAUTIFUL BACHELORETTE

EVERY SOON-TO-BE BRIDE WANTS to celebrate her last days as a single lady, but that doesn't mean she wants to look like a college student who just pulled an all-nighter, and feel even worse. Moreover, you most definitely don't want to hit rewind on all your pre-wedding-day prep! And now you don't have to.

The secret: knowing how to indulge in a way that keeps you as on track as possible, how to prevent a hangover, how to recover quickly, and how to fake it until you do.

The Bachelorette Bash Basics

This is your night (or nights!) so while you might not be the one planning all the festivities, it's important to communicate, ideally with all attendees but most definitely with your maid of honor, so you're all on the same page. Here are some things to think about and, more important, talk about, before basking in your bride-to-be fete.

THE TONE

At the end of the day, your maid of honor (or host of your bachelorette) is the one calling the shots and your job is to graciously accept the party in your honor. While there is no right or wrong way to celebrate the end of your bachelorette-hood, it is important that your girls know whether your idea of the perfect pre-nuptials party involves X-rated strippers in Vegas, a relaxing spa getaway, a low-key slumber party at a fancy hotel (complete with DIY facials, room service, and movies), a dive bar with line dancing, or any combination thereof.

THE GUEST LIST

Other than the fact that everyone invited to the bachelorette party should be on the wedding's guest list, there are no rules when it comes to invites. Whether you prefer just to party with your bridesmaids or want to include others, it's your call. Do keep your mom and future mother-in-law in mind. While they probably aren't any more interested in heading to a strip club with you than you are in having them there, if your bachelorette party is taking place at a spa or over brunch, it's appropriate to include them. And if you are planning a big (read: boozy) night out, consider inviting them to dinner and say bye-bye before barhopping.

COST

Lots of brides-to-be these days are jetting off for weekend getaways with the girls. And while this can be a blast, it's important to be sensitive to other people's budgets and to let your maid of honor (or whomever else is spearheading the party planning) know whether your priority is for everyone to be able to participate even if it means a local, low-key evening or if you'd rather go all out but know not everyone will be able to participate.

WHO PAYS

The only rule here is that it's not the bride—and that everyone knows the anticipated cost prior to accepting the invitation. Typically, each attendee pays her own way and all attendees split the cost for the bride, but it's not totally unheard of for a host to foot the bill, either, for all attendees or just for the bride.

TIMING

Anything other than the night before the big day goes. (Trust me, you do not want to look and feel hungover on your wedding day!) But for most brides-to-be, planning your bachelorette at least a month prior to the wedding will help to alleviate stress and give you ample time to recover. You also don't want to do this during the initial twenty-one Radiant Bride Detox, so plan accordingly—and ensure you have enough time to cleanse the effects out of your system before your big day.

PICTURES

Bachelorette parties can get crazy and leave all attendees in compromising positions! Consider buying disposable cameras (yup, they still make them) to safely capture all your memories and ensure they stay off-line, or just implementing a "No Social Media" rule (or, at the very least, a "No Social Media Without Prior, Sober Approval by All Pictured Parties" rule). Speaking of . . .

SOCIAL MEDIA

Whether your rule is just regarding picture sharing or anything else, make sure your girls know if there is anything you're not cool with their sharing online.

PLASTIC PENISES

There are two types of brides-to-be: those who are all about the kitschy party that's incomplete without penis-necklaces, shlong-straws, and a cock-cake and those who can't think of much worse. Same goes for the "Soon to Be Mrs." sash, faux veil, and rhinestone-encrusted crown. Figure out where you stand on this and ensure your maid of honor knows it.

STRIPPERS

See above. Same rules.

SET EXPECTATIONS

Before you and your fiancé head out on your respective night(s) on the town, it's important to discuss expectations—and a coy "don't do anything I wouldn't do" doesn't cut it. If there is anything you'd be devastated to hear your partner did, let him/her know. Also, be sure to clarify ahead of time whether you're going to share your nights' activities with each other or if you'll never talk about it again.

BE GRATEFUL

Your gal pals spent a lot of time (and likely money!) to send off your singlehood in style. Don't forget to show them your appreciation with a heartfelt note and small gift. Real beauty radiates from gratitude, kindness, and generosity so this is sure to earn you some serious beauty points!

How to Indulge Without Blowing Your Diet

You want to have fun, feel good, and party hard! Before you throw caution to the wind and celebrate your final days as a bachelorette with abandon, listen up: you can stay on track with all your bridal beauty goals and still have a boozy bachelorette party. The key: drinking smartly and preparing wisely.

Whether you're heading out to a bar or staying in with your friends, here are a few rules to keep in mind when gearing up for your last girls' night as a single lady.

LIMIT INGREDIENTS

When picking your poison, limit the ingredients (aim for a maximum of four although, in general, the fewer the better). Those sugary pre-made margarita mixes loaded with over fifteen unpronounceable ingredients? Skip them. They're what give the sweet and salty drink a bad wrap when a traditional margarita just calls for tequila, lime, and a dash of agave or Cointreau.

SKIP SODA

Between the belly-bloating carbonation and unhealthy sweeteners (whether corn syrup, cane sugar, or artificial), a healthy bride-to-be wouldn't drink soda without alcohol in it, so don't drink it tonight, either.

BE YOUR OWN MIXOLOGIST

When it comes to imbibing, not all drinks are created equal. Paired with the right mixers, your drink can help to simultaneously prevent the inflammation, dehydration, and overall dullness caused by alcohol. You just need to know the boozy bride's recipes for radiance . . . and here you have them! Whether you whip this up for a girls' night in or use them when ordering your next cocktail at a bar, you'll be beautifully boozy (and not just because everyone else is wearing their drunk goggles!).

Radiant Bride–Approved Cocktail Recipes

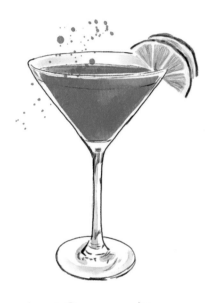

Acai Cosmopolitan

Serves 2

Tap into your inner Carrie Bradshaw with this cosmopolitan recipe that takes the *Sex and the City* favorite to beauty-boosting new heights. With acai, also known as nature's "beauty berry," this cocktail is loaded with skin-, hair-, and nail-beautifying antioxidants to help you counter the negative effects of alcohol while you drink.

---

4 ounces vodka

2 ounces freshly squeezed lime juice

2 ounces acai juice

Lime peel, to garnish

Combine the vodka, lime, and acai juice with ½ cup ice in a cocktail shaker. Shake to chill before straining into a martini glass. Garnish with the lime peel.

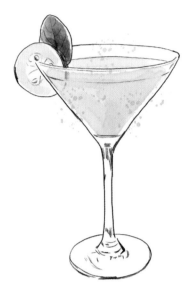

Cucumber + Basil Martini

Serves 2

Cucumber is not only super-duper hydrating, it also helps to prevent water retention. Plus, its skin, which is packed with silica, promotes skin elasticity. It's why we puree the cucumber in this recipe instead of muddling a peeled cucumber like in a traditional cucumber-based cocktail recipe!

1 six-inch piece of cucumber, seeded

6 basil leaves, divided

4 ounces gin

1 ounce freshly squeezed lime juice

In a blender, pulse the cucumber (with skin) until smooth.

Dice 4 of the basil leaves.

In a cocktail shaker, pour the gin over ice and shake until chilled. Strain and discard the ice. Return the gin to the cocktail shaker and add the cucumber puree, diced basil, and lime juice. Shake to combine before pouring into two martini glasses. Garnish with the remaining basil leaves.

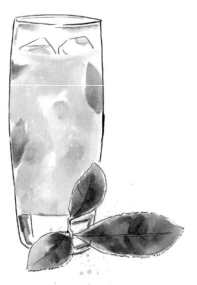

Green Tea Mojito

Serves 2

Green tea contains both polyphenols, which can decrease inflammation—including the kind that leads to pimples!—and epigallocatechin gallate (ECGC), which has been shown to boost metabolism. Combined with raw honey and mint, which are antibacterial (to fight post-party illness) and antioxidant-packed (for anti-aging benefits), respectively, and this green tea mojito will help to ensure you feel as good as you'll look!

6 to 8 mint leaves

2 ounces white rum

2 ounces freshly squeezed lime juice

8 ounces unsweetened iced green tea

2 tablespoons raw honey

Muddle the mint leaves in the bottom of a glass.

In a cocktail shaker, add the rum, lime juice, green tea, and honey. (If the honey is solid, place the honey jar in a bowl of hot water, constantly stirring until liquefied.) Add 1/2 cup of ice and shake to chill.

Pour over the mint.

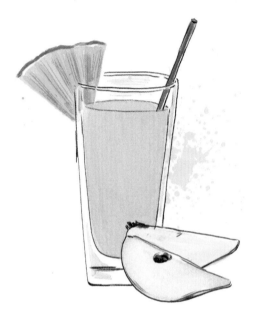

Punchy Pear + Pineapple Smoothie

Serves 2

Pears, packed with copper, potassium, iron, magnesium, and zinc—as well as vitamins C, E, B, and K!—help to promote healthy skin from the inside out. Meanwhile, pineapple, loaded with vitamin C and bromelain, an anti-inflammatory enzyme, softens skin and fights swelling. Plus, by using the whole fruit in this spiked smoothie recipe, you also get all the fiber of the fruit, which will help make you feel full, slow the absorption of both the sugar and alcohol, and prevent you from drinking too quickly! Mixed with vodka and a splash of grapefruit juice, you have the perfect fruity beverage.

3 ounces vodka

1 ripe pear, cored

1 cup diced pineapple, peeled and cored

1 cup ice

Combine all the ingredients in a blender and process until smooth. Serve immediately.

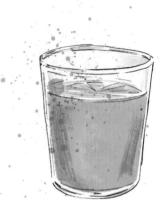

Spiked Spicy Lemonade

Serves 2

If you've ever tried the Master Cleanse, (which you shouldn't!) this may taste familiar—it's an alcoholic take on the classic cleanse drink! But that's most definitely not why I like it (and, no, sadly, this cocktail won't actually provide any detox benefits). Rather, I'm a fan of this spicy cocktail both because it's delicious and because the kick slows down your sipping and boosts your metabolism. (The capsaicin, a chemical compound found in peppers, can speed up your metabolism by about 25 percent for up to 3 hours!)

4 ounces vodka

2 tablespoon plus 2 teaspoons
    Grade B maple syrup

4 tablespoons freshly
    squeezed lemon juice

1/4 teaspoon cayenne pepper

In a cocktail shaker filled with ice, add all the ingredients. Shake to chill. Strain and divide in two glasses. Serve immediately.

How to Prevent a Hangover . . . or Recover Quickly

Let's start by making one thing clear: alcohol is processed in your body as a poison and the only way to fully prevent the harmful effects is to avoid alcohol all together. But, if you were up for that, you'd likely have skipped this section, so let's talk about lessening the evils and making sure you feel better in a hurry!

BEFORE THE BIG NIGHT . . .

STOCK UP. Whether you'll be heading home or sleeping out, stock the fridge where you'll be sleeping with everything you need to prevent a hangover: water, coconut water, and healthy snacks (especially those packed with healthy carbs and protein like almond butter and bananas!) in addition to whatever else you need in order to do all of the below.

REFRIGERATE YOUR EYE CREAM. Before you leave to go out for the night, put your eye cream in the refrigerator! When you apply it in the morning, the cooled cream will help to alleviate puffiness.

TAKE A MULTIVITAMIN. Too much alcohol can deplete your body's nutrients, so take a multivitamin before heading out to minimize the loss!

EAT. Prior to drinking (not just at 3:00 a.m. when you're already feeling crummy), eat a meal or snack with healthy fats and complex carbohydrates. Brown rice with avocado, for example, will help to line your stomach a bit and help to slow the absorption of alcohol while simultaneously providing your body with the sugars you'll soon be depleting.

WHILE YOU'RE OUT . . .

DRINK MORE . . . WATER. Alcohol is a diuretic (aka: it makes you pee!). Unfortunately, you're not just eliminating the alcohol every time you're going to the bathroom. Rather, for every ounce of alcohol you drink, your body can expel up to four times as much water. This doesn't just mean you're going to have to go to the bathroom four times more often in that gross bar bathroom, it also means your body is dehydrated, which, alcohol aside, can leave you feeling pretty crummy all on its own. The solution, drink at least one glass of water for each cocktail you drink to help fend off the dehydrating effects of too much booze.

CUT CARBONATION. Boozy bubbles not only make you bloated (a bride-to-be no-no!), but the gases may also increase the rate of alcohol absorption. Skip the carbonated mixers and, yes, even the champagne, for a more beautiful post-bachelorette morning.

STAY IN THE CLEAR. While this isn't a perfect rule of thumb, in general, darker liquors have more congeners (the other stuff produced by fermentation besides alcohol) that are responsible for a liquor's color and taste. The more congeners, the worse your hangover. Stick with clear alcohols (like vodka) and you'll feel better the morning after than if you were sipping on whisky all night.

LISTEN TO YOUR BODY. Always get a hangover when you drink sangria? Feel especially crappy the morning after margarita night? You know you best.

WHEN YOU GET HOME . . .

CHUG COCONUT WATER. Alcohol is not only dehydrating because of its diuretic effect, but also because it inhibits a hormone that keeps your body hydrated. Before hitting the sack, rehydrate with all-natural coconut water. It's rich in electrolytes and packs more potassium than a banana—making it nature's healthy alternative to the sport's drink and the ideal way to replenish your body before bed.

TAKE OFF YOUR MAKEUP. Okay, true, this may not help you feel better in the morning, but it will surely help you to look better! I know that a big bash means your nightly beauty routine will suffer, but if you do just one thing when you get home (or to the hotel), pretty please, take off your makeup. When you sleep, your energy reserves don't just replenish, your skin does, too. And if those pretty pores are covered up with makeup, your skin can't do its beautifying job. Know it will be a late night? Toss makeup-removing wipes by your bedside so you can use them without missing a bit of shut-eye.

TAKE TWO ASPIRIN. The anti-inflammatory will not only help you stay headache-free, but also will help to counteract the internal inflammation caused by alcohol, helping you heal while you sleep.

DOUBLE UP YOUR PILLOW. Grab an extra pillow so you sleep with your head more elevated than usual. It will help any retained water stay away from your face so you won't wake up with eyes puffier than ever.

IN THE MORNING . . .

SKIP THE "HAIR OF THE DOG." Myth has it that this drink in the morning will make you feel better but it's just that: a myth. The only way it helps is by numbing your senses a bit (which an Advil would do just as well) and, counterintuitively, extending the life of your hangover.

PASS ON COFFEE. It may help you feel more alert, but caffeine, like alcohol, is a diuretic and your top priority right now needs to be on rehydrating your parched body.

REHYDRATE. Sip more coconut water or puree fruit for an all-natural smoothie. The fructose will help to boost your energy levels while the fiber works like a vacuum to pull the toxins out.

DIY DE-PUFF. Dip two bags of caffeinated green or black tea in hot water to saturate them. Squeeze out the extra fluid and put the tea bags in the refrigerator or freezer to chill. When the tea bags are cool, place them over your eyes for 10 to 15 minutes to help reduce puffiness, circles, and redness; follow with your refrigerated eye cream.

SLEEP. Alcohol severely disrupts your sleep patterns. Sure, it may look like you're out like a light, but the sleep you get when drunk isn't the restorative sleep your body really needs. You may not be able to sleep well the night of your bachelorette party, but be sure to plan an easy night the next evening to help play a bit of catch up on those z's.

EAT BREAKFAST. When you wake up, load up on protein and healthy carbohydrates. It's why an egg sandwich sounds oh, so yummy the morning after.

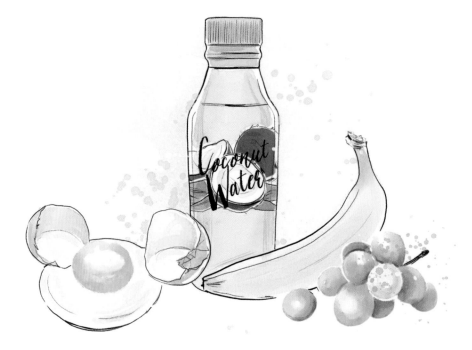

4 Hangover-Helper Breakfast Ideas

The key to eating to assuage a hangover is the combination of protein and healthy carbs. Plan ahead so you have these breakfasts ready to go the morning after. The best part: they're all dairy- and gluten-free and part of your Radiant Bride Diet! (Of course, don't eat anything that doesn't typically agree with you.)

P.S. Feel free to share this with your maid of honor. I feel a bridal breakfast in bed in the works!

Breakfast Quinoa Bowl

Serves 2

Packed with super-healthy and easy-to-digest protein and all your essential amino acids, this is one of my favorite go-to breakfasts no matter the prior night's festivities.

1 cup cooked quinoa, prepared according to package instructions

2 tablespoons raw almond butter

2 tablespoons raw almond slivers

1/4 cup canned chickpeas, rinsed and dried

1/4 cup raisins

1/3 cup raw hemp seeds

Sea salt, to taste

Combine all ingredients in a mixing bowl. Divide and serve.

Quick Tip

Prepare ahead of time and keep it in the fridge for a hangover-helper breakfast that's ready when you are!

Gluten-Free + Sugar-Free Granola

Serves 4

I like to make a big batch of this and keep it in my freezer in smaller portions that I can pop out the night before for use in the morning.

3/4 cups gluten-free rolled oats

1/4 cup raw pistachios, shelled

2 tablespoons raw pumpkin seeds

2 tablespoons raw sunflower seeds

2 tablespoons raw pecans

2 tablespoons raw walnuts

2 tablespoons raw almonds

2 tablespoons raw cashews

3 tablespoons unsweetened shredded coconut

2 tablespoons cinnamon

1/2 teaspoon salt

1/2 cup cold-pressed coconut oil

Preheat the oven to 350°F.

In a large bowl, combine all of the dry ingredients. Add the coconut oil and stir until coated.

Spread the mixture evenly on a parchment-lined baking sheet. Bake for 40 minutes, stirring at 10-minute intervals to prevent burning.

Serve with almond milk, if desired—or just eat it straight out of the oven!

Quick Tip

Make this recipe up to 4 months before and store it in the freezer. Remove it the night before you head out and surprise your guests with a home-made breakfast the morning after your girls' night! Best part: you can bring the granola and almond milk with you anywhere and order ice to chill the almond milk and spoons from most room service menus!

Potato Scramble

Serves 2

While the carbs will satisfy your hangover craving for something solid, it's the eggs here that really deserve all the credit. Loaded with cysteine, they basically act like a sponge, soaking up the toxins your bachelorette bender left behind.

2 teaspoons olive oil, divided

4 small red potatoes, cubed

1 leek, diced

1 teaspoon diced thyme

4 eggs

Salt and pepper, to taste

In a large sauté pan, combine the olive oil, potatoes, and ¼ cup of water. Cover and cook for about 5 minutes longer than it takes to bring to a boil, or until the water has evaporated.

Uncover and sauté, constantly stirring, until the potatoes begin to brown, about 5 to 7 minutes. Add the leek and thyme.

In a small bowl, scramble the eggs.

Add the eggs to the potatoes and stir until the eggs are cooked to your liking. Season, with salt and pepper, if desired, and serve immediately.

Quick Tip

You can cook the potatoes the day before and just reheat them before sautéing with the eggs. Also, don't be shy with the salt. It will help your body to retain water and rehydrate more quickly—and we can blast the bloat come Monday!

Vegan + Gluten-Free BLT

Serves 2

Craving a sandwich come morning—or, like any good New Yorker, a bagel with egg and cheese? Make this vegan and gluten-free take on the BLT instead and you'll satiate your craving while staying firmly on your wedding diet track!

½ avocado

2 slices gluten-free bread, toasted

4 slices smoked tempeh

2 iceberg lettuce leaves

¼ tomato, thinly sliced

Mash the avocado until smooth. Spread half of the mashed avocado on each half of the toasted bread. Top one half with the tempeh, lettuce, and tomato. Cover with the second piece of bread. Slice in half and serve immediately.

⟨ Quick Tip ⟩

Ensure you have all of the ingredients prepped ahead of time and all you'll have to do is toast and assemble come morning. Not vegan and up for cooking? Add an egg prepared over hard to the sandwich for even more hangover-healing protein.

FAKE IT: How to Hide the Signs of One Too Many Cocktails

Whether you're meeting your fiancé for brunch or just would prefer not to look like death even within the confines of your own home, look like a million bucks (even if you feel like trash!) with these beauty-boosting and hangover-concealing tips. And for all you ladies on a multi-night bachelorette weekend, this is so you can rock it on night two looking as fresh as ever!

GET CLEAN

You'd be surprised how many "under circles" are primarily residual eye makeup leftover from the night before! Before you start fretting and concealing, clean your face one more time (let's be honest, last night's beauty routine wasn't exactly up to par). Have stubborn eyeliner, mascara, or glitter (hey, no judgments!) stuck in place? Dip a cotton swab in coconut oil or olive oil to gently and effectively remove even the most stubborn makeup without irritating your eyes.

REHYDRATE

Your skin is one of the first places to show the signs of dehydration (and few things dehydrate you more than alcohol or a sleepless night) so any hangover beauty routine needs to start with some serious hydration, both from the inside out and outside in. Step 1: chug some water—or, better yet, coconut water, which is packed with hydration-boosting electrolytes, too. Step 2: apply moisturizer to that clean face of yours.

DE-PUFF

If you have an extra white potato lying around, apply thin slices to your eyes for ten minutes. Potatoes not only retain their chill for longer than cucumbers, but also contain catecholase, an enzyme used in pricey eye creams, that reduces the appearance of under eye circles! No potatoes around? Place anything cold on your face. Even two spoons popped in the freezer for a couple of minutes can do the trick.

EVEN OUT

Late nights leave even the most even-skinned among us blotchy and dull. To give yourself a boost without caking on the makeup, DIY your own ultra-brightening BB cream: mix equal parts of your favorite foundation with your usual day cream before adding a dab of luminizer. Apply all over your face and follow with concealer, as needed. If you're feeling queasy, add some powder to prevent any clamminess from showing through.

BLUSH

Add a dab of cream blush to the apples of your cheeks (the part that puffs out a bit when you smile). The creamy consistency will help add a vibrant (not clammy!) dewiness to your complexion for a youthful, fresh finish.

HIGHLIGHT

Just as a bright yellow highlighter grabs your attention when used in books, highlighting with makeup will do the same for your face and, when used strategically, help to conceal the signs of a sleepless night. Dab a bit of golden or cream shimmer to the innermost corners of your eyes and on your brow bone to make your eyes look more awake, and add a soft swipe to your cheekbones to make your skin appear radiant.

CURL

Not your hair. Your lashes. Just a quick clamp of the eyelash curler (don't worry, with a bit of practice you'll be a pro in no time) and you'll immediately look more awake. Follow with waterproof mascara and your makeup is good to go!

REDO THE 'DO

Sure, a shower will make you feel better, but if you couldn't resist hitting snooze and run out of time, or are just hoping to salvage a picture-perfect blowout from the night before, dry shampoo is your new BFF. Spray sparingly to your roots. Use your fingers to rub it in for instant volume and oil coverage. Hair still looking bed-head-like? Use bobby pins (or a Goody Spin Pin, which is my favorite!) to secure hair in an elastic-free bun. In a few hours, undo the 'do for runway-ready waves, painlessly.

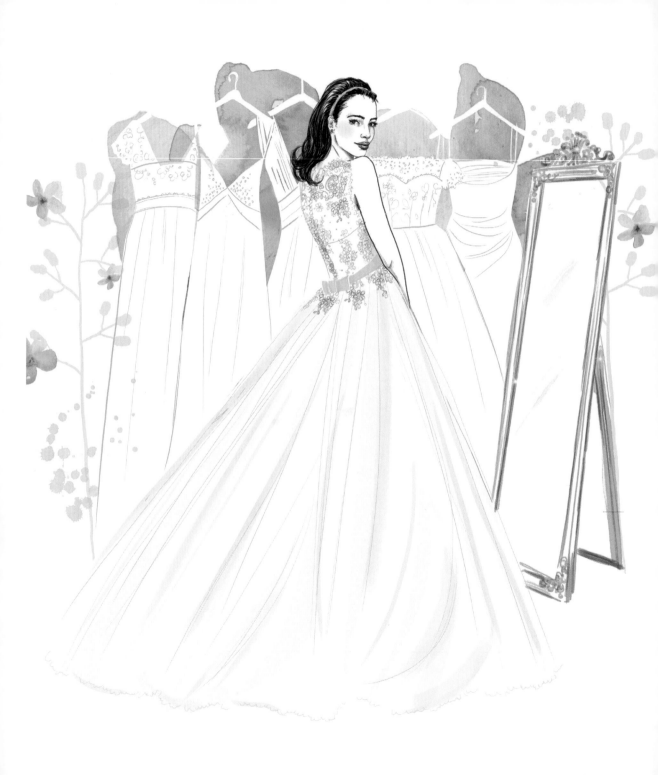

Chapter Five

PICKING THE PERFECT DRESS(ES)

YOU WANT TO FIND *THE* DRESS—the one that makes you look and feel like everything you've ever imagined. Heck, the average woman spends approximately $1,200 on her wedding dress (and many, many women spend much, much more than that!), making this not only a huge investment in a piece of clothing, but also, for many women, a large chunk of the wedding budget. Needless to say, it's important to get this right!

While flipping through magazines is a great way to garner inspiration, just as jeans and blouses may look great on mannequins in store windows, but not quite right on your body, wedding dresses, too, may look beautiful on a model in a magazine or on a hanger in a store, yet not on your body. It's all about finding the right dress for you—your body, your skin tone, your taste, your budget, and your personality—and I'm here to help with some general guidelines to make this exponentially easier and ensure you feel (and, yes, look!) your best.

Let me start by saying I *hate* the fruit-as-body-type classification system far too many fashion pros rely on to help you find your best look. Not only are we all uniquely shaped, but we also all feel differently about our fruity shape (one "pear" may want to flaunt her sultry curves while another wants to do everything she can to conceal them), making any type of body shape-based guide extremely limiting.

I couldn't care less what fruit you (or I) resemble. I just want you to feel amazing on your wedding day! So, instead of focusing on your body type and telling you what works best, here are the most popular wedding dress silhouettes, necklines, and sleeve styles, with insider tips designed to help you navigate an overly saturated wedding dress market that can be overwhelming at best and panic-attack provoking at its worst.

But just remember, these are only guidelines, so take it all with a grain of salt as you tap into your inner seven-year-old and relish in playing dress-up. You'll know you've found your perfect dress when you try it on and feel like a million bucks.

Selecting the Silhouette

If you're unsure where to start, deciding on your favorite silhouette is the easiest way to narrow down your choices. Referring to the general shape of the gown, the silhouette is, for most brides, the first thing they think of when imagining their dream dress.

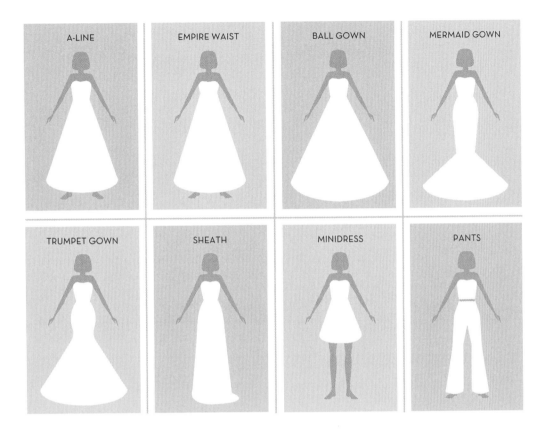

A-LINE

With a flare beginning at your natural waist line, this universally flattering style slightly hugs your torso before flaring out in a shape reminiscent of the letter A. It's especially great for women who don't want a full-on ball gown but nevertheless want to slightly conceal their hips/thighs/bum, while still showing off their upper body. If you feel overwhelmed with the options or lost as to what you want, this is a pretty safe place to start your search.

Celebrity Inspiration: *Kate Middleton, Jennifer Lopez, Ivanka Trump, Jewel*

EMPIRE WAIST

If you want to show off your chest or really conceal your waist, try an empire style. With a fitted chest and a skirt that begins to flare from right under the bustline, this is not only one of the most forgiving dress styles, but also one of the most customizable since the shape of the flare can vary from relatively straight to A-line, allowing you to control how much of a gown you're up for. This is also the ideal style if you're pregnant since it easily accommodates a growing bump.

Celebrity Inspiration: *Liv Tyler, Jennifer Garner*

BALL GOWN

With a bodice fitted like the A-line but paired with a very full, dramatic skirt, this style is ideal if you're self-conscious about your large bust, since it not only draws the eye down, but also balances out typically top-heavy proportions. It's also great for women really wanting to have their princess moment.

Celebrity Inspiration: *Jacqueline Kennedy Onassis, Kim Kardashian*

MERMAID GOWN

If you have curves and don't want to hide them (you shouldn't!), the mermaid dress is for you. Fitted throughout the bodice and flaring out at the knee (or lower), the mermaid dress is form-fitting throughout and oh so sexy. It's not, however, very forgiving. If you're on the shorter side, have the flare begin just above the knee to elongate your silhouette.

Celebrity Inspiration: *Brooklyn Decker, Mariah Carey, Hilary Duff*

TRUMPET GOWN

Similar in shape to the mermaid, but both less dramatic and more flattering for many, the trumpet gown shows off your chest, waist, and hips with a body-skimming shape, before flaring out just below the hips.

Celebrity Inspiration: *Fergie, Beyoncé*

SHEATH

This slim, straight style typically skims the body from chest to hips before falling straight to the floor. This is especially flattering for women with an athletic build or those not feeling the princess look.

Celebrity Inspiration: *Carolyn Bessette-Kennedy, Kate Moss*

MINIDRESS

For brides getting married beachside, a short dress can be the practical choice, although it's also great for brides getting hitched in-land looking for more dancing freedom (or just to show off those toned legs!). It's also become a popular choice for brides looking to change their outfits either between the ceremony and the reception or between the reception and the after party. Just be sure two dresses are *really* in your budget before getting your heart set on a mid-night outfit change.

Celebrity Inspiration: *Cindy Crawford, Yoko Ono, Keira Knightley*

PANTS

Yup, I said it: just because everyone is telling you to wear a wedding gown, they're not for every-one and your wedding is *yours*! Hate dresses? Don't wear one! For a still bride-like-look, wear wide leg pants in white or ivory or take inspiration from Olivia Palermo and wear tailored shorts with a sheer skirt overlay.

Celebrity Inspiration: *Ellen DeGeneres, Olivia Palermo*

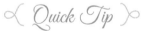

Quick Tip

For the bride who wants to get down on the dance floor without worrying about stepping on her dress (and for whom a second, shorter dress isn't of interest or in the budget), most of these silhouettes can be made tea-length (ending between calf and ankle) for more mobility—and to show off those new shoes of yours!

Nailing the Neckline

⬦

From modest to plunging, the neckline of your dress is as important as the silhouette in creating your look. It's also a great way to adjust the feel of a silhouette that on its own may not be the most flattering for your body. Use these neckline guides to help find the right style to help draw attention away from wider hips, or to enhance what nature may or may not have given you.

BATEAU

This relatively high neckline cuts straight from shoulder to shoulder, elongating the neck and making shoulders appear wider. This will help to emphasize a small waist and balance wider hips, but isn't best for women with already broad shoulders nor the bride who wants to be able to dance the night away.

OFF THE SHOULDER

Revealing more skin than the bateau, but with a similarly straight across neckline, this sexy but classy style broadens the shoulders, giving the illusion of a more cinched waist (even on a sheath silhouette). It's an ideal way to add drama to an otherwise simple gown and is also perfect for showing off a statement necklace. It can constrict your dance moves though, so be mindful of that before committing.

HIGH COLLAR

Either in the fabric of your gown or in a sheer lace, a high neckline adds some serious runway-like drama to any silhouette. Ranging from a mock turtleneck height to the entire length of your neck, a high collar pairs beautifully with sheer lace sleeves as well as if your religious ceremony requires a more conservative style but you prefer a bit of sass. Just beware busty ladies, it can draw additional attention to your already accentuated assets, distracting from the rest of you and your dress.

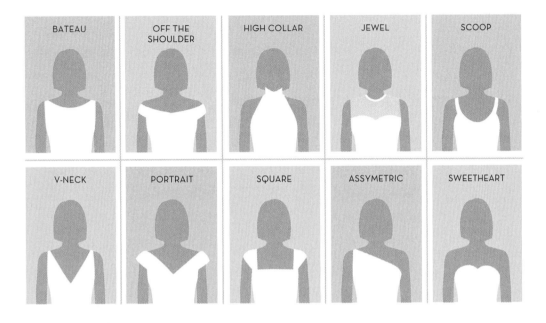

JEWEL + SCOOP

Clean and classic, these universally flattering rounded necklines may seem simple, but they perfectly complement dramatic skirts and intricate fabrics. They also provide a large amount of flexibility with regard to where you'd like to fall on the modest-to-sexy spectrum since they can cut as high as the collarbone (otherwise called the jewel) and as low as you'd like to go (the scoop).

V-NECK + PORTRAIT

Like the jewel and scoop, the differentiating factor between the V-Neck and Portrait is the shape of the V. Where the portrait is a wide, shallow V running from shoulder to shoulder often revealing only the smallest amount of cleavage, if any, the V-neck, conversely, is typically much deeper and more revealing, though not as wide. While both are stylistically similar, the V-neck elongates both the neck and chest and flatters wide shoulders, while the portrait makes shoulders appear broader, ideal for balancing wider hips.

SQUARE

Most commonly seen on strapless dresses, the straight across style is universally flattering so long as it's paired with the right strap or sleeve option. (Women with broad shoulders, for example, should pair it with a strap to help give the illusion of a narrower silhouette.) Paired with a cap or short sleeve, the square neckline can also be used to add modern right angles to a simpler silhouette.

ASYMMETRIC

For the trendier bride, an asymmetric neckline can allow you to add a bit of personality to your gown, without compromising on sophistication. It's especially flattering on small to medium busts, although with the right fabric and cut, this can work on anyone!

SWEETHEART

If you're less well-endowed up top and want to create the illusion of a larger chest, this is the neckline for you! Not only because the style gives the illusion of curves, but also because it's easily enhanced with a built-in padded bra—just ask your dress shop to sew your favorite one inside.

Considering the Sleeves

No matter your chosen silhouette and neckline, your sleeve choice can dramatically alter the overall look and feel of your gown, making any style appear more romantic, conservative, sexy, or dramatic.

STRAPLESS

One of the most common styles (and for good reason!), this classically sexy look is flattering on most body types. Just be careful the dress fits your bust perfectly both so it doesn't dig into you, giving the illusion of unflattering armpit fat, and so you're not constantly adjusting yourself throughout the night. And don't forget to jump around a bit before committing to ensure you can dance the night away without worrying about a nip-slip! A great tailor should be able to sew in the right underpinnings so even the bustiest of women can confidently bare all.

SPAGHETTI STRAP

If you have broad shoulders or a large chest, a spaghetti strap will allow you to show lots of skin while breaking up your shoulders (making them appear narrower) and offering more support to a larger bust.

WIDE STRAP

Like with a spaghetti strap, wide straps (which can be anywhere from half an inch to a few inches) are a great way to de-emphasize broad shoulders or a large chest. They're also ideal if you want to show off toned arms. Arms not your favorite feature? Skip the wide strap and instead choose a sleeved option.

HALTER

Available in any strap width, from spaghetti to wide, a halter style can help give a beachy, more casual vibe to any dress.

CAP + PETAL

This small shoulder cover not only broadens the shoulders (ideal for women with wider hips) but also adds a bit of classic, conservative glamour to any gown. The difference between the two: the cap sleeve is more structured while the petal sleeve is softer and more flowy.

SHORT SLEEVE

From a fitted T-shirt style to a flowy flutter, a bellowing balloon to a romantic Juliet pouf, a short sleeve on a wedding gown can help take attention off your chest, make a dress more conservative or less formal, or just add a bit more style to a simple gown. The more volume the sleeve has, the broader it will make your shoulders and the narrower it will make your waist, so keep that in mind when picking a style.

THREE-QUARTER

Ideal for daytime weddings and any bride looking to conceal less than toned arms, this style is universally flattering (although it's much more popular with older brides).

LONG-SLEEVED

Having made a big comeback since Kate Middleton donned a lace long-sleeved style, this regal sleeve can take many forms, but all add some serious drama. To keep it classic, try a slim, fitted sleeve in the same fabric as your dress, like Grace Kelly. For a sexy take on sleeves, try a fitted illusion sleeve in a stretchy, sheer fabric or lace. For more toned arms, look for a more simple lace, while less toned arms look best in a more intricate lace. For added drama, try a bell sleeve (like bellbottom pants but on a sleeve), a poet sleeve (fitted from shoulder to elbow before bellowing out and cinching again at the wrist), or a leg-of-mutton (bellowing from shoulder to elbow and fitted from elbow to wrist).

Picking the Perfect White

Tradition may call for white, but most brides today—yes, even those committed to tradition—are steering away from the stark shade and instead picking a hue closer to ivory or champagne. And for good reason! Stark white isn't especially flattering on most skin tones (it can make you look washed out) but that doesn't mean you still can't revel in your white-like moment. The key: picking the most flattering shade for you.

Quick Tip

Every designer has their own names for the colors of their fabrics so pay less attention to the name and more to your own assessment of the hue.

WHITE

A true white is most flattering on women with dark skin and cool undertones. Not sure whether you have cool undertones? If you look better in silver than in gold and blues and purples flatter you more than oranges and corals, you're likely cool. But a stark white, no matter how cool your undertones, will still always look better on darker skin.

OFF-WHITE

A slightly creamier shade than white, but not quite as warm as ivory, this shade works on most skin tones (although women with olive skin should look for an off-white with more yellow than pink undertones for the most flattering shade). If you're set on "wearing white" but know stark white isn't the most flattering shade for you, this is a great place to start.

IVORY

This creamy shade is also flattering on most skin tones and an especially great choice for fair-skinned brides. Like off-white, ivory can have yellow or pink undertones, so make sure to try on a few different ivory gowns to ensure the most flattering hue.

CHAMPAGNE

A bit warmer than ivory, with yellow undertones, this shade looks great on women with similarly warm undertones to their skin. If you're a bit olive (no matter how pale or dark your skin) and look better both in gold than silver and corals and orangey reds than cool blues and purples, this is a great choice.

OTHER SHADES

Sure, white may be tradition, but that doesn't mean it's for you. Not into a white gown? Cool! Sarah Jessica Parker famously wore a black wedding gown, Gwen Stefani and Christina Aguilera rocked pink ombré gorgeously, and Julianne Moore wore a lilac sheath. Just make sure you think it through and make sure you won't later be disappointed in having missed out on the white dress moment. And don't forget the option of adding a satin belt in another hue to your dress to give it some individual flare (you can add it on just for the reception, if you prefer, as well).

The Veil

It's considered an accessory, but when you walk down the aisle, it's one of the first things anyone will notice, making it pretty important in my book! From a vintage-inspired birdcage to a voluminous pouf, from a heavily embellished cathedral to a simple waterfall, your veil can—and should!—be a showstopper, so you don't want it to merely be an afterthought.

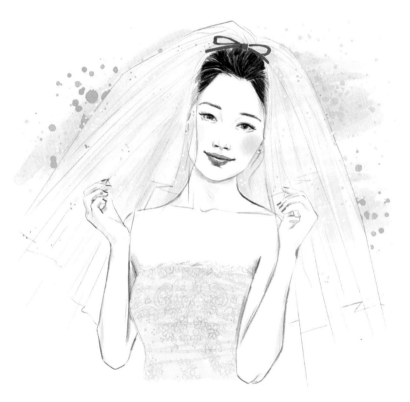

COVERAGE

Traditionally, veils were designed to veil the bride's face. Today, there are few steadfast rules when it comes to bridal fashion and the veil is no exception. Consider whether you want to wear a veil at all and, if so, whether you want it over your face or just to cascade down your back.

LENGTH

Wherever your veil ends, the eye will be drawn, so make sure that's a place you want to emphasize. A veil with trim will have an even more obvious end point, making this an exponentially more important consideration, while a veil with cascading edges will have a less eye-catching end. As a general rule, you don't want your dress and veil to end at the same point, so either choose a veil considerably shorter than your train, or have it continue a few inches past the train of your dress.

VOLUME

A full veil will add volume to your face, which is great if you have a long, narrow face, but not if your face is rounder. Similarly, a long, flowing veil will soften and elongate your face, making it ideal for rounder and more angular faces.

Quick Tip

You'll want to remove your veil after the ceremony (or, at the very least, right after the first dance), but if you want to keep the headpiece or hairpin it's attached to on for the reception, make sure it's removable on its own via hooks or even Velcro.

Your Underpinnings + Lingerie

Not that you should skip the gym (don't you want to be radiantly healthy for decades to come?) but if there's one thing that can help you fake a flawless figure, it's underpinnings. From all-in-one body shapers to cinchers, bras to petticoats, having the right undergarments can be the difference between looking drab and feeling fab.

It's especially important to select your undergarments for your wedding day ASAP since they will not only affect how your dress looks (and how sexy you feel!) but also how your gown fits and the alterations required. If you're not 100 percent sure what will work best, buy a few options and bring them all to your first fitting (other than underwear, most underpinnings are returnable, but be sure to double-check).

BRA

Depending on your gown's structure and your bust size, a bra may not be necessary. If it is, ensure the straps are perfectly concealed and/or ask your tailor to secure the bra in the dress so you don't have to worry about the straps peeking out. As for color, a nude bra will be your best choice for a seamless appearance, but if it's not sexy enough for you, aim for a white that matches the lining of the gown. And you wouldn't believe how many of us are actually walking around in the wrong bra size so now would also be a great time to get a professional fitting so your bra doesn't cause any unwanted lumps and bumps due to an improper fit (most major department stores have fitters on staff).

SLIP

A slip will make all dresses lay more smoothly. One with some elastic in it can actually work as a full body-support stocking, sucking in any and all unwanted bulges! Again, you want this to either match the color of your skin or the color of your dress's lining for a perfectly finished look. If you're wearing a slim-fitting dress, be sure to find a seamless slip so it lies invisibly underneath. Even you super fit ladies likely want a slip to ensure your dress glides over your body effortlessly.

CORSET OR CINCHER

Often thought of as the stereotypical bridal lingerie, the corset (or more modern and less constricting cincher) is often seriously structured and full of boning (which I like to think got its name from its bone-poking proclivity). While a corset or cincher can pinch in your waist and emphasize your curves, keep in mind that you'll be wearing your dress for numerous hours and don't want to be uncomfortable. It can also give you a stomachache. Heart set on the look of the cincher? Wear it around your house for a few hours before committing.

PETTICOAT

Like a tutu worn underneath a skirt for added volume, a petticoat is an essential part of both ball gowns and dramatic A-line wedding dresses. Custom and couture gowns that require a petticoat typically have one already built into the garment, but if you would like to wear a second one for additional fullness or if your gown doesn't come with one (but needs it), make sure you buy it before you begin your dress fittings since it will shorten the skirt.

HOSIERY

Although generally unnecessary under gowns (and inappropriate with open-toed or backless shoes), if you are going to wear hose, give yourself some piece of mind and buy a few extra pairs to cover yourself in the event of a run.

GARTER

While both the bouquet and garter tosses are wholly optional (and, yes, you *can* do one without the other!), and many brides today are forgoing this tradition, a lot of brides choose to wear a garter as their "something blue." Just be sure it is invisible under your dress and that it stays up (so you're not fidgeting with it) and is invisible. And if you are planning on tossing your garter, buy a second one to save!

DON'T FORGET TO . . .

Consider comfort. *Think about the ease with which you'll be able to dance when trying on a dress. Sure, some styles have serious wow factor, but when it comes to enjoying your night, you want to be able to comfortably do everything you want to do!*

Look behind you. *Pay attention to the back of your gown. It's what most guests will be looking at during the ceremony.*

Learn how to bustle. *Especially if your gown has a long train that's not removable, ask your maid of honor to come to one of your fittings in order to learn how to bustle your gown, so you don't step on it all night long.*

Add a pocket. *Ask your seamstress to add a small, invisible pocket to your gown, if possible, so you can keep lip gloss on hand for touch-ups!*

Pay it forward. *Think about donating your dress after your wedding to a not-for-profit or selling it yourself and donating the proceeds.*

Look close to home. *Ask your mom if she still has her veil. It's a great "something borrowed!"*

Buy a dress that actually fits! *Some women think the smaller the garment they squeeze into, the smaller they'll look—but the truth is that stuffing yourself in a size that's too small will just cause unflattering lumps and bumps.*

Something Blue:
9 New Ways to Marry in Blue

1) In the lining of your dress, ask your seamstress to sew a small blue ribbon, bow, or feather.

2) Embroider your wedding date and/or new monogram on the inside of your dress in blue thread.

3) Have your stylist invisibly secure a blue bobby pin to your hair or look for a hairpin with blue stones and incorporate it in your style.

4) Paint your toenails in a light blue.

5) Wear blue underwear. Just make sure it's invisible under your dress.

6) Incorporate blue blooms in your bouquet.

7) Sapphires add regal elegance to any wedding gown.

8) Paint the soles of your shoes blue for a subtle pop of color.

9) Have your seamstress swap out a layer of white tulle with a light blue one.

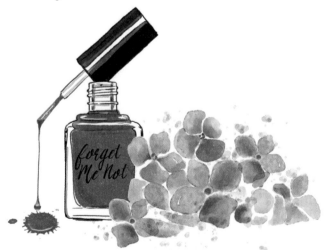

Shopping + Fittings 101

Heading out in search of your dream dress? If you embark prepared, the process will be easier for all parties involved!

BRING PICTURES OF WHAT YOU LIKE. And what you don't like, for that matter, so the person helping you at the store can see which silhouettes, necklines, sleeves, and shades of white, most interest you.

WEAR THE RIGHT UNDERPINNINGS. If you've already found your dream dress and are going in for fittings, wear the undergarments you'll wear on your wedding to ensure everything looks perfect. On your first shopping trip? Remember that at the very least the person helping you— and potentially your bridal party, your mom, and future mother-in-law included—will see you in your underwear. Today's not the day to wear your raciest lingerie.

BRING THE SHOES YOU WANT TO WEAR. If you haven't yet bought your wedding shoes, bring something you own with a similar heel height. This is essential for fittings in order to determine the proper length, but it's helpful even for the first round of shopping.

BRING A SNACK. Dress shopping can be surprisingly exhausting. Some raw nuts or dried fruit can be a lifesaver!

WEAR MINIMAL MAKEUP. You don't want to risk getting makeup on the dress!

BRING COMPANY. A second set of eyes (ones you trust, of course!) can be priceless.

ASK FOR A FABRIC SWATCH. While most wedding salons know the importance of lighting, it's nevertheless important to look at your fabric in other lighting sources, so ask for a swatch you can look at outdoors, at home, etc.

BRING A CAMERA. Not all places allow you to take pictures, but if they do it will be enormously helpful—not only to share with your BFFs but also to show your florist and cake designer, who can use your dress as inspiration. Just make sure your betrothed doesn't see it accidentally!

Your Bridesmaids + Maid of Honor

This day is all about you, but that doesn't mean your bridesmaids (and their dresses) don't deserve some TLC (even if only for the selfish reason that you want your pictures to look amazing). Been dreaming of a lime-green, strapless-dress donned bridal party? Before you outfit your ladies in a hue sure to wash some of them out—and potentially reflect poorly on you—here are some things to keep in mind.

THE STYLE

Just as no one style of a wedding gown or shade of white looks good on every bride, no one bridesmaid dress style looks good on every one of your friends. Sure, a traditional wedding calls for some degree of cohesiveness, but instead of outfitting all your nearest and dearest in an identical dress, it's far more modern to consider similar rather than the same. Consider picking a general color (navy blue, for example) or shade of colors (blush tones, for example) and letting each of your bridesmaids choose her own gown (just ask for them all to be the same length). Not only will your bridesmaids be more comfortable—and thereby look more beautiful—they'll also look better in your pictures. Or, if you're set on your wedding party being dressed alike, head to a store that sells a wide selection of bridesmaid dresses and choose a few similar dress styles in the same color and fabric and let your attendants pick the most flattering for her body. Your ladies in waiting—especially those with less easy-to-fit bodies—will be very grateful.

Really have your heart set on all of your bridesmaids dressed in the same exact gown? Bring as many of your attendants shopping with you as you can to help you in choosing the most flattering fit.

Quick Tip

Your bridesmaids' dresses should be ordered three months before the big day to allow for delivery time and alterations.

THE COLOR

Standing next to your nearest and dearest clad in chartreuse? Not only will the hue likely wash many of them out, it will also reflect on you—both bouncing off your white dress, giving it a slightly yellow hue, and off your skin, giving your face a sickly tint. If you're set on all your bridesmaids in matching dresses, the most universally flattering hues are black, chocolate brown, and deep jewel tones, like emerald green, amethyst purple, and sapphire (navy) blue, which will not only ensure they look radiant, but that you do, too.

Quick Tip

If all of your bridesmaids are to be dressed in the same fabric, encourage them all to place their orders at the same time in order to ensure each dress is cut from the same dye lot, to prevent any subtle color differences.

THE ACCESSORIES

Another way to create cohesiveness among bridesmaids in different dresses is to have each of your attendants wear the same broach, sash, or statement necklace. This works especially well when bridesmaids are all in varying tones of the same color family—and doubles as a great bridesmaid gift too!

Dressing all your attendants alike? Don't forget to give them ample notice of any special requests regarding accessories. But if all your bridesmaids are in the same or even similar gowns, allowing some flexibility on jewelry, shoes, and handbags will be much appreciated.

Consider adding the same sash your bridesmaids are wearing (or a sash in the same color as their dresses) to your gown after the ceremony. It will add a bit of colorful flair to your gown for the reception and give the illusion of an outfit change, too.

Quick Tip

Instead of a more traditional wedding party gift, consider paying for your bridesmaids' dresses. They've likely already spent a lot of time and money on your special day, and if your budget allows for this, they'll be incredibly grateful.

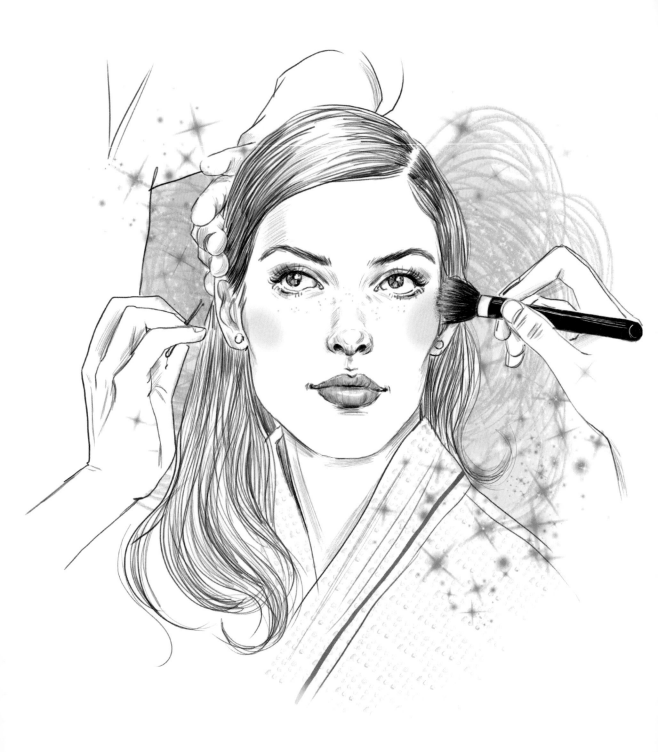

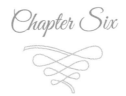

Chapter Six

BEAUTIFYING THE BRIDE

I'VE NEVER MET A BRIDE-TO-BE FOR WHOM looking and feeling her most beautiful on her wedding day wasn't the ultimate goal from the moment the ring hit her finger. Yet far too many women focus so much on their diet and fitness and completely ignore their skincare, makeup, and hair until mere days before the wedding when they're suddenly relying on a last-minute glam squad to take their skin from dull to dynamite and their hair from flat to fab. And, sadly, there's only so much even the most incredible makeup artists, facialists, colorists, and hairstylists can do in such limited time. The ball's in your court, lady, and I'm going to show you how to play the game.

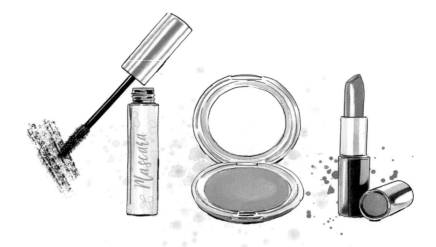

The Beauty Cleanse: Out with the Old

Most women have a medicine cabinet, drawers, or closets stocked with products . . . but oftentimes, none of the right ones. Now is the time to toss the old and restock your beauty arsenal with the products you need to be your most radiant self on the big day. Here is my guide to the insider secrets and DIY tips to keep you glowing from engagement to happily ever after.

This may be tough—especially if you're the beauty-obsessed type—but trust me here: old makeup and skincare products, like medicines, have expiration dates—not merely because active ingredients expire, products dry out, and colors go out of style, but because products (especially those kept in your steamy bathroom) are the prime place for bacteria to set up shop. Plus, you need to get rid of the old (to make room for the new, of course). So get out a trash bag (and some tissues, if you sense tears brewing) and let's get started.

MASCARA + LIQUID EYELINER

Once it's been opened, toss it after three months. Once air gets into the formula, the consistency starts to change and preservatives start to break down, leaving you susceptible to eye infections.

FOUNDATION + CONCEALER

While they can last up to a year if you consistently apply them with a clean applicator, if you use your fingers, a brush, or sponge that's anything but spanking clean, they should be tossed every six months. If you notice the layers separating in your liquid foundation or the color changing, it's definitely time for it to go. Plus, your skin tone changes seasonally, so every six months it's a good idea to reevaluate your shade, too.

FACIAL CLEANSERS, LOTIONS, + CREAMS

If they have SPF or are in a tub or pot in which you place your fingers to apply, they should be tossed after six months. SPF's efficacy begins to diminish after six months, and fingers in cream are like a bacteria swingers' party. If they're SPF-free and have a pump dispenser, they can last up to one year.

CREAM MAKEUP

Once opened, toss them after six months. If unopened, it will depend on the brand (or, more accurately, how many preservatives the brand uses), so look for changes in color or consistency to determine whether to toss.

POWDER MAKEUP

Every twelve to eighteen months, go through all your powdered cosmetics and chuck them to prevent your skin from looking dull or breaking out, and your makeup from flaking off. Makes you reconsider buying sixteen eye shadows at once, huh?

LIPSTICK

If you regularly dip it in alcohol to sanitize it, it can last up to two years, but if it looks dried out, it's time to let go.

LIP GLOSS

Every year they have to go. Toss sooner if you notice it's stickier than usual—or if you regularly leave them in your hot car.

LIP LINERS + EYELINER PENCILS

If they can be sharpened (in a clean makeup sharpener!) and dipped in alcohol each month, they can last eighteen to twenty-four months, although if you have an eye infection at any time, toss eyeliners immediately.

MAKEUP BRUSHES

High-quality, well taken care of makeup brushes can last practically forever (it's one of the things most worth investing in when it comes to your makeup). It's essential, though, that you keep them clean! You wouldn't use the same washcloth to wash your face for months on end, so don't do the same with your brushes. Shampoo them weekly in baby shampoo and warm water and lay them on a clean towel, with the handle slightly elevated (so gravity helps pull moisture to the ends of the bristles), to air-dry overnight.

ALSO!

Toss anything if you notice a change in smell, color, or consistency. Keep products fresh longer by ensuring that all packaging is closed tight and stored in a cool, dry place (like a refrigerator or linen closet). And never share makeup—even with family members!

In with the New: Restocking Your Stash

Now for the fun part: restocking your now likely bare beauty bag! Regardless of your skin type and budget, these are the products you should stock to keep your skin clean, clear, and protected; the essential information you need to make informed decisions when shopping; and the details on how to best use all these goodies.

FACE WASH

Whether you wear makeup daily or prefer to go *au natural*, washing your face every evening before bed is a must to remove pore-clogging and aging environmental pollutants. If you have dry or sensitive skin, look for a cleansing oil that will break down and wash away dirt and grime, while maintaining your skin's delicate moisture barrier. If you have very oily or acne-prone skin, look for a foaming cleanser with salicylic acid to help break down the sebum that's clogging your pores. And if you ever even think about going to sleep without washing your face, pick up a pack of makeup removing wipes to keep by your bed. They won't replace the need for facial cleanser, but they're better than nothing once in a while. Unless you have very oily skin, you can skip washing your face in the morning (or just splash some water on it if you like).

EYE MAKEUP REMOVER

If you're wearing eye makeup, it's essential to have an eye makeup remover—and not just to prevent looking like a raccoon come morning. The skin around your eyes is especially thin and prone to damage (that's why it is often the first place to show signs of aging), so it's essential to treat the area with a bit more TLC. Plus, you need to keep your eyelash follicles clean and clear in order to promote eye lash growth—and we all want longer, thicker eyelashes! I like to use pure extra-virgin cold pressed coconut oil to gently remove my eye makeup (I dip a cotton swab in the coconut oil, gently rub it on my eyes, and repeat until the swab is clean), but there are a lot of drugstore brands that will do the trick. The key is to find something that's easy to use and to use it very gently.

DAY CREAM

No matter your skin type, you need a day cream. It's the type of day cream you need that varies. If you have oily skin, the goal is to add water-based hydration to your skin so your body recognizes it's adequately hydrated and stops overproducing pore-clogging sebum. If you have dry skin, you need to add both water and oil back into your skin for balance. To add water to your skin, look for a product with hyaluronic acid. This superstar skincare ingredient can retain up to 1,000 times its weight in water, bringing serious hydration deep within your skin. If you have very oily and acne-prone skin, a gel-based moisturizer with hyaluronic acid is best, since it will add moisture back into your skin without increasing the amount of oil. If you have combination or dry skin, use an argan, olive, or coconut pure oil, or oil-based lotion on top.

SPF

If your day cream doesn't have SPF, find one you love and apply it regularly. It can be a cream, powder, or in your makeup but nothing keeps your skin looking its best better than avoiding sun damage, so make sure to apply it thoroughly and to reapply often. Yes, even if it's rainy or over-cast—and don't forget your neck and décolleté. If you have skin prone to breakouts, try a BB cream, which will help keep skin clear while also providing sun protection—and even light coverage!

NIGHT CREAM

Just as your brain rejuvenates as you sleep, so, too, does your skin, which is why products applied before bed are so effective. Regardless of your skin type, if you're over the age of thirty or prone to breakouts or age spots, look for a moisturizer with retinol to help encourage cell turnover. Under thirty and generally have great skin? A few drops of coconut or argan oil warmed between your hands and gently pressed on your face will do the trick!

EYE CREAM

It's the first place to show the effects of sleepless nights and the earliest signs of aging. If your primary concern is under-eye puffiness or circles, look for one with caffeine as an active ingredient. More worried about fine lines and wrinkles? Look for peptides, hyaluronic acid, vitamins C and E, and retinol (if your skin can tolerate it).

EXFOLIATING SCRUB

Feel free to just add a tablespoon of white sugar to your facial cleanser and scrub that way, or to buy an exfoliating scrub. If you're buying one, just make sure that it uses nuts, seeds, or sugars as the exfoliants, not salt (which dehydrates skin), apricot kernels (which are very popular, but are too harsh for your facial cells), or microbeads (which are bad for the oceans). Use it two to three times per week at the end of a warm shower, when your skin cells are loosened.

ANTIOXIDANT SERUM

The best way to prevent changes in skin texture and tone over time is to arm your skin cells with an army of troops trained to fight all the environmental elements aging your skin. An antioxidant serum is just that. Look for one with vitamin C as its primary ingredient and apply it every morning on a clean face.

SPOT TREATMENTS

If you have acne or dark spots, you should have a targeted product designed to treat just that issue. Sure, an acne-targeted face wash is great and a CC cream designed to even skin tone is lovely, but when you really need some targeted attention, look for a product designed *just* for that. For hyperpigmentation, look for something packed with vitamins A and C.

For acne, look for something with tea tree oil to naturally kill bacteria and dry out blemishes—or pull out the big guns with salicylic acid or benzoyl peroxide, although the Sahara-like conditions they typically create can lead to more breakouts down the road.

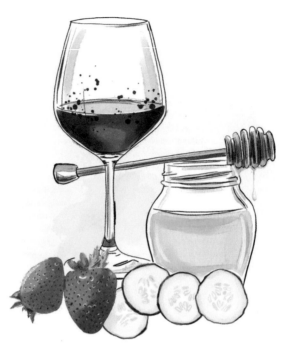

4 DIY Facial Masks

◇

Once or twice a week, treat yourself to an at-home facial to target your skin's primary concerns. DIY it with an all-natural homemade facial recipe you can make with ingredients you likely already have in your kitchen. You can buy facial masks, too, but the active ingredients in food are actually more effective (and better for your skin) so if you can, whip up one of the recipes on the next few pages. Really prefer not to DIY it? Look for masks with limited ingredients, targeted for your exact skincare needs.

Gentle Chemical Peel

Let fruit acid in the strawberries and lactic acid in the yogurt help to gently break down the dull, dry skin cells fogging your complexion. Then, scrub it all away with sugar to reveal a brighter, dewier complexion (perfect for flawless makeup application).

For dull, dry, clogged skin, not for very sensitive skin

2 medium strawberries	*Puree the strawberries in a food processor until smooth.*
2 tablespoons full-fat Greek yogurt	*Mix the strawberry puree and yogurt until well combined.*
1 tablespoon white sugar	*Apply a thin layer to your face, neck, and décolleté. Let dry for twenty minutes before using the sugar to exfoliate the mask off. Rinse with warm water.*

Anti-Aging Hydrating Face Mask

The vitamin A–packed egg yolk helps to encourage cell rejuvenation and the red wine bathes your skin in free-radical-fighting antioxidants, while the honey helps to pull moisture deep within your skin. The result: soft, smooth, supple skin that looks and feels younger.

For dry or aging skin

1 egg yolk	*In a small bowl, beat the egg yolk. Slowly add the wine and honey, stirring constantly to mix. Apply to your face, neck, and décolleté with a pastry brush, avoiding your eyes and lips. Let dry for 15 to 20 minutes before washing off with your favorite facial cleanser.*
1 tablespoon red wine	
1 tablespoon raw honey	

Blemish-Busting Facial Mask + Spot Treatment

Yogurt, with its probiotics to balance bacteria and lactic acid to break up clogged pores, is one of the best blemish fighters around. Combined with vitamin A–packed sweet potato to help encourage cell turnover and antibacterial honey, this mask quickly and painlessly reduces redness and inflammation without drying out your skin.

For acne-prone skin

---

2 teaspoons plain Greek yogurt (at least 2 percent milk fat)

1 teaspoon sweet potato puree

1/2 teaspoon raw honey

In a small bowl, combine all ingredients until smooth. Apply a thin layer to affected areas and let sit for 20 minutes before rinsing off with warm water. You can use this as a daily spot treatment, too.

Calming Cucumber Latte Compresses

The caffeine in the coffee constricts your blood vessels to reduce redness, while the cucumber calms your skin, and the milk promotes healing.

For red or irritated skin

1-inch sliced cucumber, with skin

2 tablespoons caffeinated coffee

1 tablespoon whole milk

Combine all ingredients in a blender.

Refrigerate to chill.

Saturate cotton rounds in the mixture and apply to affected areas until no longer cool. Repeat for 10 minutes before rinsing your face with cool water.

Makeup Musts

When it comes to stocking a makeup bag, you really don't need much so long as you have the correct tools. Here are the musts.

CONCEALER: Make sure it's a match with your skin type and tone and that you have two different ones: one for under your eyes (to correct blues) and one for blemishes (to correct reds).

LUMINIZER: This can be in a stick or pot and comes in varying levels of creaminess, but you want something that's very subtly shimmery and slightly golden that you can use to make your eyes appear more open (by dabbing it on the inner corners of your eyes), to highlight your cheekbones or brow bones, to highlight the bow of your lip, or even to make your nose appear thinner (by running a thin strip down the center). It can even double as eye shadow.

BRONZER: Add a swipe of healthy glow to your skin all year round, without the harmful effects of the sun. The younger you are, the more shimmer you can get away with. Over forty? Shimmer settles in fine lines and wrinkles, making them appear more pronounced, so be cautious, especially around your eyes.

BLUSH: A flushed cheek makes everyone look just a bit healthier and happier. Look for a sheer pink shade that you can build up for more coverage or barely swipe on for less.

MASCARA + EYELASH CURLER: Make your eyes appear larger and more awake, instantly, with a quick clamp of an eyelash curler and a swipe (or two!) of mascara. Look for a tubular formula with flexible polymers, which literally create tubes around your lashes for greater volume and length without the risk of flakiness or difficulty taking it off. Warm your lash curler by running it under hot water for an even more dramatic curl.

LIPSTICK, LIP GLOSS, TINTED LIP BALM: It's all about preference here. Have fun and experiment to find you signature shade.

Makeup Maybes

———◇———

Depending on your personality, you may want these, too!

EYELINER: When you're looking especially tired, lining the inner edge of your lower lash line helps conceal the redness that gives away the signs of a sleepless night. When you want to add drama, play with the thickness of your liner on your upper lid.

FOUNDATION: For medium to full coverage of very discolored skin, try foundation. If you have acne-prone skin, be sure to look for a foundation with acne-fighting or calming ingredients like green tea or salicylic acid. For all skin types, make sure it has SPF, too.

BB CREAM: If you have acne-prone skin and are looking for light to medium full-facial coverage, try a BB cream instead of foundation. It's designed to not only conceal acne but also to help treat and prevent breakouts.

CC CREAM: Uneven skin tone got you down? CC creams, a color-correcting, anti-aging and foundation hybrid, will help to even your skin tone immediately and over time help to correct the discoloration.

TINTED MOISTURIZER: For light coverage without any skincare benefits, look for a tinted moisturizer (or just mix a few drops of foundation with your day cream to DIY it).

EYE SHADOW: It's essential for any sort of a dramatic eye, but for every day, your bronzer, blush, and luminizer can get the job done.

PRIMER: If you have oily eyelids, at the very least you'll want an eye primer to help keep your eye shadow from creasing. If you have oily skin, or are prone to sweating off your makeup, a face primer is a good idea for you, too.

Body Care

Your skin is exponentially less sensitive from your head to your toes, so if you can only restock one portion of your beauty stash at a time, start with your face and work your way down.

BODY WASH/SOAP: If your skin is very dry or sensitive, be sure to buy a non-foaming moisturizing formula since those sudsy bubbles can strip your body of its natural oils. Prone to breakouts? Look for an acne-fighting body wash with salicylic acid.

BODY LOTION: Your skin is your body's largest organ and body lotion gets applied to most of it so look for all-natural formulas, or just pick up a tub of coconut oil at the grocery store and use that.

ANTI-CELLULITE SCRUB: There's a joke that 90 percent of women say they have cellulite, and the other 10 percent are lying. Odds are: you have it, too. For an over-the-counter solution, look for both a scrub and a cream with caffeine as an active ingredient. To DIY it, use coffee grounds to temporarily reduce the appearance of cellulite, practically for free!

Anti-Cellulite Coffee Scrub

This exfoliating scrub has vitamin E–packed wheat germ oil to promote healing and caffeine-loaded coffee grounds to increase circulation and reduce the dimpling effect.

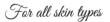

For all skin types

1/2 cup cooled, **caffeinated coffee grounds** 1/4 cup **wheat germ oil**	*Combine the coffee grounds with the oil in a small plastic bowl. In the shower, use your hands to scrub cellulite-ridden skin in vigorous circular motions for 5 to 10 minutes. Rinse clean. Repeat daily.*

Hair Care

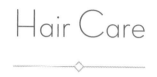

Your hair may be dead, but that doesn't mean it doesn't need its fair share of love and attention!

SHAMPOO: Sulfates strip hair of its natural oils, making dry hair drier and oily hair oilier (since it throws your body's oil-production mechanisms into high gear), so you'll want to avoid those. Look for formulas specifically designed for the type of hair you have and the type of hair you want. And regardless of your shampoo, remember to just wash your scalp and let the shampoo run through the lengths of your hair. There's no need to suds up the lengths of your hair when all it does is dry it out.

CONDITIONER: Again, look for formulas designed both for the type of hair you have and the kind you want. Opposite of shampoo, only put conditioner on your hair, not on your scalp, to hydrate the lengths of your tresses without weighing down you locks or clogging the pores on your scalp.

STYLING PRODUCTS: Depending on how you like to style your hair, look for products designed just for that. If you're using heat tools, make sure to use a protecting spray before use to save your strands from frying. Struggling with frizz? Apply serums from the mid-lengths of your hair to the ends, but avoid the roots. Have flat hair? Try spraying dry shampoo through all your hair from root to end to give texture and volume to even the most flat manes. (If you have dark hair, look for tinted formulas to avoid a powdery finish.)

DEEP CONDITIONING MASKS: Once a week, apply a hydrating mask to towel-dried hair to help repair damage and replenish your strands. If you color your hair with anything containing red or warm browns, beware: the red molecule seeps from your hair shaft far more easily than any other hue, so make sure your mask is designed especially for color-treated hair. And if you see red water washing down the drain, use the mask only every other week to preserve your shade.

DIY Hydrating Hair Mask

Hydrate dry hair and repair damaged strands with this nutrient-packed hair mask designed to prevent breakage, split ends, and dullness.

For all hair types

1 ripe avocado

1 egg, room temperature

2 tablespoon coconut (at room temperature) or olive oil

In a small, plastic bowl, mash the avocado until smooth. In a separate bowl, scramble the egg. Mix the avocado, egg, and oil until well combined. Apply the mixture to towel-dried hair from root to end. (If you have very oily hair, avoid your scalp.) Cover with a shower cap and let sit for 10 to 15 minutes before shampooing out. Style as usual.

HOW TO EXTEND THE SHELF LIFE OF YOUR BEAUTY PRODUCTS + STAY ORGANIZED

Find storage space. *Whether it's a shelf in a linen closet or even in your fridge, find a cool, dry, dark place you can store your makeup and skincare products. A mini fridge in your bathroom is the ultimate luxury, but even a dresser drawer will do, so long as your beauty products are not in a hot, steamy bathroom.*

Buy a caddy or bag. *If you're going to keep your makeup and skincare products outside of your bathroom (and you are!), you're going to need to make it as easy as possible to get them where you need them, so make sure you have an easy to carry bag or caddy.*

Get cleaning tools. *You'll need baby shampoo to wash your makeup brushes, alcohol to dip your lipsticks, lip liners, and eye liner pencils in, and a makeup sharpener to sharpen anything that can (and should) be sharpened regularly.*

Picking Your Wedding-Day Hair + Makeup

With both your makeup and hair, the key to looking like the best version of yourself on your wedding day is to wear your hair in some variation of your usual hairstyle and your makeup in the same ballpark as you usually do so you feel the most comfortable and "like you." If your hair is always down and straight, now is not the time to try ringlets pinned in an updo, even if your hairstylist insists it will look great. (It may, but when you look at your pictures you won't think it looks like you.) Same goes for a red lipstick if you're really more of a nude gloss kind of girl.

Really set on trying something new? Just make sure you try it ahead of time, more than once, and wear it around a bit to make sure you really love the look.

WEDDING HAIR STYLES TO FLATTER YOUR FACE SHAPE

Torn on how to wear your hair or what style will be the most flattering? Start here!

If Your Face Is Round . . .

An asymmetrical style will be the most flattering. Start with a deep side part to elongate your face before pulling your hair off to one side in a low ponytail, braid, or bun. If you want to wear your hair down or are set on a center part, have your stylist cut long layers, with the shortest layer hitting at or below your collarbone.

Want a center part and an updo? Make sure the bulk of your hair that's up is secured higher up on your head than the top of your ears, and without too much volume (like in a sleek ponytail), for the most flattering look.

If Your Face Is Oval . . .

A center part with volume, either with hair down or pulled back, is the most flattering. Bangs also look great on you, although if you don't already have them, don't risk hating them with a cut now.

If Your Face Is Square . . .

Add loose waves at the ends of your hair to bring softness to the angular shape of your face and create a center part to draw the eye down the center of your face, away from the broadness of your jawline.

If Your Face Is Heart-Shaped . . .

A style that ends at chin or neck length (like a low, voluminous bun or long bouncy bob) will help to add volume to the lower half of your face, softening the triangle shape. Alternatively, a deep side part will help to narrow your forehead. Want to wear your hair down? Long layers with the short-est falling between your chin and collar bone will help to fill in the area around your chin.

WEDDING-DAY MAKEUP TIPS

PRACTICE MAKES PERFECT. Like with most things, practice goes a long way with your makeup, especially if you're doing it yourself. Not only will it help you to perfect your skills, it will also help you to gauge how you need to tweak your everyday makeup for your wedding so that it wears and photographs best. For the best results, wear a shirt in the same color as your dress when you're practicing (so it will help you to see more clearly how you'll look when donning your gown) and ask a friend to take some pictures of you in various lighting conditions to see how your look will photograph.

TEST YOUR EYE MAKEUP UNDER VARIOUS CONDITIONS. You don't need to wear your full bridal face makeup around town or to the office, but you should wear your desired eye makeup a few times to test and ensure it doesn't flake or run throughout the day.

CONSIDER THE CLIMATE. If you're getting married in a hot climate, use mattifying and/or oil-free products to help diminish unwanted sheen.

USE A PRIMER. On your face and your eyes, a primer will help to ensure your makeup stays in place all day long.

DO YOUR EYES FIRST. If your eye shadow falls onto your cheeks (which it will!), you won't have to redo your face makeup.

PUT ON FOUNDATION BEFORE CONCEALER. Foundation will often take the bulk of redness out of a blemish or the majority of blue out from under your eyes, limiting the need for concealer and keeping your makeup from looking cakey.

USE DIFFERENT CONCEALERS. The best concealer to cover blemishes or other facial redness will have a green undertone while one that covers blues will have yellow undertones. Make sure you have one for each.

MIND YOUR BROWS. They frame your face, especially in pictures, so don't forget to use brow gel and to fill them in, as needed.

CONSIDER FALSE LASHES. They may look silly in their packaging, but they photograph beautifully. Just make sure to test them out plenty of times beforehand to ensure your eyes aren't sensitive to the glue or weight of the lashes. You should also experiment with various styles to find the most flattering ones for you.

KEEP IT SIMPLE. I know I've said this already, but don't go overboard. Sure, a smoky eye looks pretty in magazines, but if you've never worn it before, you may feel uncomfortable on the big day and you may not like your pictures in the future. The best wedding makeup leaves you looking like you at your prettiest, not like someone else.

Your Beauty Calendar Countdown: From Today to 30 Days to Go

6+ MONTHS
BEFORE THE BIG DAY

LOAD UP ON BEAUTY VITAMINS. If you want to jump-start your skin and hair's rejuvenation process, make sure you're getting enough of your beauty vitamins for longer, shinier hair and glowing skin. The essentials: iron, protein, B vitamins. Not getting enough in your diet? Talk with your doctor about taking supplements. They take at least three months to start showing their effects so start early and stick with them.

EXPERIMENT. Thinking about trying a new hair color or cut? Be sure to do it at least six months before the big day so if you hate it, there's ample time for your hair to grow out or to fix a dyesaster.

START LASER HAIR REMOVAL. If you're planning on embarking on a hairless journey, now is the time to start since it takes multiple sessions before you start seeing results and you need to wait at least four weeks between sessions.

STICK WITH YOUR SKINCARE REGIMEN. If you have problem skin (including facial-acne, body-acne, or rosacea), consider consulting a pro to discuss the best treatment plan, which may include laser treatments or facials to help jump-start your skin's healing process.

4+ MONTHS
BEFORE THE BIG DAY

TEST SELF-TANNERS. If you want to experiment with self-tanners, now is the time to start to perfect your technique or to find a professional you can trust.

BOOK HAIR + MAKEUP. Make appointments both for trial runs (for four weeks before the big day) and for the day of your wedding with your beauty glam squad. If you're getting married in a new city, call either the hotel you're staying at on your wedding night (or the nicest hotel in town) and ask to speak with the concierge. They usually know all the best people around. (More details on what to bring and ask in Chapter 7). If you're not hiring a pro, visit a makeup counter at a department store for a makeover (make sure they know exactly the look you're going for) and purchase anything you need now so you have plenty of time to practice your wedding day makeup. Bring a friend along for moral support—or just so you're not talked into buying a random purple eye shadow!

3+ MONTHS
BEFORE THE BIG DAY . . .

GET YOUR BROWS PROFESSIONALLY SHAPED. If you've never had your eyebrows professionally shaped and you want to do it for your wedding, try it for the first time now so you'll have time to grow them out if needed. You'll have them done again closer to the wedding, too, so they look perfect on the big day. Remember: subtle grooming is always best!

2+ MONTHS
BEFORE THE BIG DAY

FINALIZE BEAUTY ACCESSORIES. If you're going to wear a hair adornment or don a custom lipstick shade, figure that out now.

TAKE YOUR FITNESS TO THE MAX. Really focus on toning those muscles of yours! If you have been procrastinating on your workouts, now is the time to really dive in.

GET A FACIAL. Use an at-home facial mask (see pages 114–116) or book a salon facial. You will relish in the relaxing downtime and your skin will have sufficient time to calm down in the event of developing redness. Don't forget to let your facialist know of any allergies and that you're getting married so she keeps it gentle.

READY FOR YOUR
30 DAY COUNTDOWN?
READ ON!

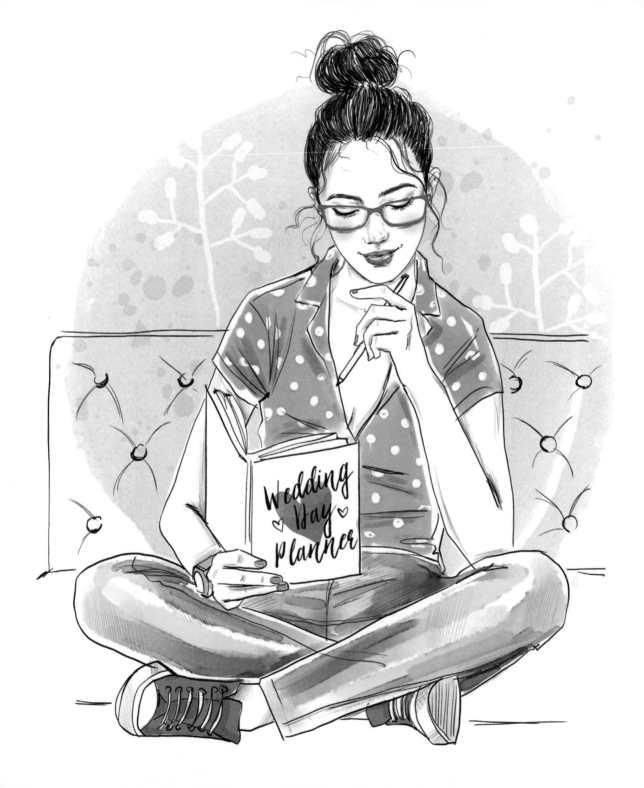

Chapter Seven

30 DAYS TO GO

IT'S CRUNCH TIME AND YOU'RE STRESSED OUT.

Don't be.

I'll help you through the home stretch!

The Appointments You Need to Make NOW

———◇———

Some things you can DIY (body scrubs). Others you should outsource (bikini waxes!). And some are all about preference and budget (facials, massages, etc.). To ensure you don't get stuck begging your colorist to stay late to touch up your roots before the big day, ensure all your outsourced appointments are scheduled well in advance so you can beautify stress-free.

First thing first: you need to decide whether you want to spend full days taking care of all your wedding-day beauty appointments, or if you'd rather spread it out over the course of the month. While this will largely depend on your schedule—and that of your glam squad—it will also depend on whether you'd prefer to spend a full day glamming it up (exponentially easier if the appointments are in close proximity to one another), or if you prefer to spread the beautifying cheer over the course of evenings after work, for example. Or some combination thereof. Once you decide on your desired plan, pick up the phone and start making these appointments—the sooner the better.

SCHEDULE FOR **4 WEEKS BEFORE** THE BIG DAY

○ *Final dress fitting*
○ *Makeup trial run*
○ *Hair trial run*
○ *Professional teeth whitening, if desired*

SCHEDULE FOR **2 WEEKS BEFORE** THE BIG DAY

- ○ *Hair trim*
- ○ *Hair color touch-up*
- ○ *Eyebrow shaping*
- ○ *Gentle hydrating facial*
- ○ *Facial waxing*

SCHEDULE FOR **1 WEEK BEFORE** THE BIG DAY

- ○ *Body waxing (legs, bikini, under arms, etc.)*
- ○ *Massage*

SCHEDULE FOR **3 DAYS BEFORE** THE BIG DAY

- ○ *Gels, acrylics, or gel polish*

SCHEDULE FOR **2 DAYS BEFORE** THE BIG DAY

- ○ *Spray tan, if desired*

SCHEDULE FOR **THE DAY BEFORE** THE BIG DAY

- ○ *Manicure, if desired*
- ○ *Pedicure*

SCHEDULE FOR **THE DAY OF**

- ○ *Makeup*
- ○ *Hair*

10 Questions to Ask Your Hairstylist + Makeup Artist Before Booking

———◇———

1) What is your fee and payment policy? If required, is there an additional fee for travel?

2) How much time do you anticipate needing?

3) Will you stay on hand throughout the day/night for touch-ups—and, if so, is there an added cost?

4) If not, will you provide me with products for touch-ups? Or are there products I should buy in advance to do touch-ups myself?

5) Do you bring your own products? Am I responsible for providing anything?

6) What kind of space and lighting do you need?

7) Will you style my bridesmaids? If so, how much additional time do you need and what will be the added cost?

8) Will you be bringing an assistant?

9) How should I prepare on the big day? Should my hair be wet? Should I apply my skincare products?

10) Do you have references and/or pictures of brides you've styled recently?

4 Weeks to Go . . .

With a month to go, it's the time to do all the beautifying things that can be done in advance. Get as many of these out of the way to free up your schedule as the big day (quickly!) approaches.

HAVE TEETH WHITENED, IF DESIRED. If you're getting your teeth professionally whitened, do it now to avoid teeth sensitivity and allow the white streaks that can show up after an in-office treatment to fade. (Don't worry, they're a temporary result of dehydrating your teeth.) If you're going to use a store-bought whitening strip system, start using them now since they often take multiple uses to reach the desired shade.

DO YOUR MAKEUP + HAIR TRIAL RUN. If you're having your hair and makeup professionally done for your wedding, go in now for a test run to make sure you and your beauty team are on the same page. Have your makeup artist write down everything used on a face chart so you have a record of it handy for the big day and take lots of pictures for your hairdresser to reference the day of as well. And don't forget to bring your veil or headpiece for the hair trial.

　　If you're having a destination wedding and are unable to schedule a test run with the makeup artist and hairstylist who will do your hair and makeup on the big day, consider buying all the products used during the test run to bring with you so you'll be able to more easily replicate the look when you arrive at your destination. For more complicated hairstyles and makeup applications, consider asking your maid of honor to come and videotape the trial run so you can either share it with the team at your destination or DIY it. Make sure to time how long it all takes, too, so you can plan your day-of beauty routine accordingly.

HAVE YOUR FINAL DRESS FITTING. Schedule your final dress fitting about four weeks out from the wedding. Make sure you bring all your undergarments and accessories to test them, too.

MEET WITH THE PHOTOGRAPHER. Discuss the look and feel you want for your pictures and the people you want to ensure are photographed most. Show him or her photographs of you that you love so he or she can see how you prefer to be shot. You can do this via e-mail or over the phone, too, if you're not in the same city.

EXFOLIATE. Soft skin is a marriage must. If you haven't already, start exfoliating your body with a hydrating scrub two to three times a week. Make sure to use a sugar-based scrub, as salt can further strip your skin of moisture.

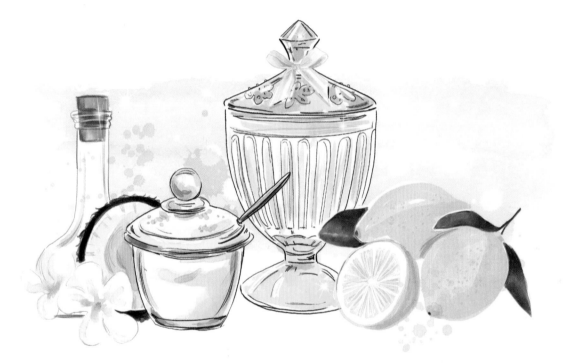

DIY Hydrating Body Scrub

This scrub contains lemon juice to help loosen dead skin cells. With its citric acid, two different kinds of sugar to manually exfoliate (white sugar for a more fine exfoliation and sugar in the raw for a deeper scrub), and coconut oil for its deeply hydrating properties, all dead, dull, dry skin cells making your skin appear ashy will be a thing of the past.

½ cup white sugar

½ cup sugar in the raw

2 tablespoons fresh squeezed lemon juice

½ cup coconut oil, liquefied

Combine all ingredients together in a plastic bowl.

After a warm shower to soften your skin, use your hands to scrub your body from chest down in circular motions. Use a washcloth for a deeper scrub on the thicker skin around your feet, knees, and elbows.

Rinse with warm water, leaving the oil to moisturize throughout the day.

Repeat 2 to 3 times a week.

GRADUALLY SELF-TAN, IF DESIRED

Considering a self-tanner? Try a gradual one instead! With four weeks to go, you'll have plenty of time to start using a daily lotion with gradual tanning properties (available at any drugstore). The results may not be as immediately dramatic, but you'll eliminate the risk of streaks and random dark spots. Hey, you know what they say: slow and steady wins the race (they may as well have been talking about self-tanner).

Also—now would be a good time for me to remind you that tanning booths are *never* a good idea!

2 Weeks to Go . . .

Take care of all the things you want to do as close to your wedding day as possible, while still leaving plenty of time to deal with any potential disasters (like redness from a facial or a haircut you hate).

GET ANOTHER GENTLE FACIAL. If you like professional facials, now is the time to go in for your last one. This should be a facial that you've had before, with an esthetician you've used before. You should also let your esthetician know your wedding is approaching and that you don't want her to try anything new (and risk an adverse reaction). If you prefer to DIY it, do a facial recipe you've used before. If you can't squeeze in a facial this week, skip it rather than having it any closer to your wedding.

TRIM YOUR HAIR. No experimenting here, either, just stick to the look you love and have it freshened up. Ideally, you'll do this exactly two weeks before the big day—leaving enough time for your trim to settle in while remaining fresh—but, if you must, you can do this closer to the wedding so long as it's with your regular stylist and he or she knows the stakes!

TOUCH UP YOUR HAIR COLOR. This is the time to freshen up base color, touch up roots, or add shine with a gloss. Don't try anything new—not even subtle highlights your stylist swears will brighten your face (they might, but if you want to try them, do it at least a month before the wedding or wait until after the honeymoon).

HAVE YOUR EYEBROWS SHAPED. Have your brows professionally shaped by your favorite eyebrow expert for the last time before the big day. I can't emphasize this enough: don't try anything or anyone new. If you have fast-growing hair, you can schedule this five to seven days prior to your wedding, although I'd still rather you tweeze stragglers a few days before the wedding than risk redness or irritation too close to the big day. If you wax other parts of your face, do so now as well.

INCREASE YOUR CARDIO. Not for the burn, but for the endorphins and stress release! Your body and soul will thank you.

CONFIRM DAY-OF BEAUTY APPOINTMENTS. Call to confirm your makeup, hair, and nail appointments.

PICK OUT YOUR NAIL COLOR. Decide on what nail color you'll wear. If you're getting gels, call to confirm your manicurist has your desired shade in stock. If you're getting a traditional polish manicure, buy your preferred polish color ahead of time both to protect yourself in case your salon runs out of the shade and so you'll have the exact same hue available for touch-ups in case of a day-of chip. Two bottles of the same "color" can be slightly off if they're from different batches so use the same bottle on your nails that you'll have on hand for touch-ups.

PRACTICE DOING YOUR OWN HAIR + MAKEUP. If you're planning on doing your own hair and makeup, practice this week to ensure you're both comfortable and happy with the results. Time how long it takes you to help gauge how much time you'll need the day of.

1 Week to Go . . .

This week is all about taking care of business, and trying to relax, too!

BODY WAX, IF DESIRED. If you want to be hair-free for the honeymoon lingerie, now's the time to wax so your skin has time to calm down in the event of any irritation or redness. If you have sensitive skin, or just want to take an abundance of caution, ask the esthetician to use hard wax (which is gentler) and to double-check the temperature of the wax to prevent any unintentional burns. Immediately apply a cortisone cream afterward to help further prevent redness and bumps.

SPLURGE ON A MASSAGE. If you have any room left in your budget, schedule a couples massage for you and your fiancé—boy, do you both likely deserve it! Not in the budget? Pull out the kitchen timer and some coconut oil and give each other a thirty-minute massage.

DEEP CONDITION YOUR HAIR. Use your favorite deep-conditioning treatment for softer, shinier hair. Cover it with a shower cap and wrap it in a hot towel for added hydration.

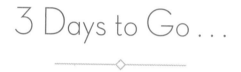

3 Days to Go . . .

Ensure your skin radiates with a gentle at-home treatment, and get long-wear nail treatments out of the way, if possible. The next few days are going to be busy so try to relax.

DO A GENTLE AT-HOME PEEL. While a professional chemical peel is too harsh to do only a few days before your wedding, if you've been using the facial peel recipe from page 115 and know your skin responds well to it, schedule time to DIY now. It's not merely relaxing, but will also leave your makeup-free skin glowing and ensure a more even makeup application.

GET GELS, ACRYLICS, OR GEL POLISH. If you're going for any of these kinds of manicures, consider scheduling it now. If you're taking off from work the one to two days before your wedding and have more time then, there's no harm in waiting, but this is something you can get out of the way three days before (during your lunch break or after work!), to give you more time for the rushed days ahead!

2 Days to Go . . .

It's crunch time and you're likely feeling anxious, excited, and a bit nervous. Everything you're feeling is normal and to be expected but now's not the time to let nerves get the best of you!

SCHEDULE A WORKOUT. Whether you're DIYing most of the party planning and feel like there's too much to do and not enough time, or you're leaving it all in the hands of a party planner and just waiting to show up, plan time to hit the gym today. The endorphins will energize and relax you—and, I've never heard anyone say they regretted exercising!

TOUCH UP YOUR BROWS. Only if absolutely necessary, use tweezers to carefully clean up any stray hairs that fall well outside the perimeter of your brows. *Do not* tweeze more than the few sparse hairs that may have popped up since your professional shaping. This isn't the time to reshape your brows; rather this is just for plucking away outliers.

GET A SPRAY TAN OR USE SELF-TANNER. If you're going to go for the faux glow, schedule your spray tan or plan to DIY it two days before the big day to give the tan time to fade in and look more natural—and to prevent tanner from staining your dress. Do not, however, try a new tanning product or technique before the big day. You don't want to risk looking Oompa Loompa orange!

HOW TO APPLY SELF-TANNER FLAWLESSLY

◆ *Don't wait until the big day to try out self-tanning for the first time. Start practicing months before to ensure you're happy with the results and have your technique down pat!*

◆ *Exfoliate beforehand with an oil-free scrub or, even better, an exfoliating mitt, loofah, or towel, to help the self-tanner to absorb evenly.*

◆ *Avoid using deodorants or perfumes prior to tanning, as they can leave a residue that leads to an uneven tan.*

◆ *Wear gloves to avoid unnaturally tanned palms.*

◆ *Put a light layer of lotion on dry spots (like knees, toes, and elbows) to avoid dark patches.*

◆ *Keep damp cotton swabs nearby and immediately wipe self-tanner from sunspots or old acne scars, which tend to get darker and more noticeable with self-tanner.*

◆ *Start from your feet and work your way up to avoid unintentional tan lines caused by bending over.*

◆ *Remember that less is more. You can always apply another coat.*

◆ *Wait at least eight hours before showering.*

◆ *Too dark or uneven? Alternate rubbing the cut half of a lemon and a warm washcloth on areas that are too dark or streaky until faded.*

◆ *Want to clean it all off? Buy a self-tan removing product or, if in a bind, soak in a bubble bath for about twenty minutes before using an exfoliating scrub or gloves to scrub it away.*

1 Day to Go . . .

—◇—

You're in the homestretch, beauty! Now, it's all about the details.

SHAVE. If you're going to shave (rather than wax), do so today so that in the event of a cut, you have plenty of time for it to stop bleeding before putting on that dress of yours. It will also give you a day to spot any missed spots you can touch up tomorrow, if needed.

GET POLISHED. If you're going with a traditional polish mani/pedi, schedule it for today because a) you're not going to be patient enough to sit on your wedding morning and b) you want to minimize the time between polish and vows to reduce the risk of chips.

SCHEDULE "ME TIME." Schedule time to do something that relaxes you. Draw yourself a bubble bath (do this *before* your mani/pedi!), take a long walk, or pop into your favorite yoga studio. Or just schedule some alone time with your fiancé so you can connect. The only rule: you can't talk about the wedding.

DRINK LOTS OF WATER. Your energy levels and skin will thank you.

GET YOUR BEAUTY SLEEP. The best thing you can do at this point is to at least try to get some z's. Even if you can't sleep, get into bed, close your eyes, and just try to shut off your mind and rejuvenate your body. To up the beautifying powers of your shut-eye, try to sleep on your back with your head slightly elevated to prevent fluid from accumulating under your eyes, making you appear drowsy.

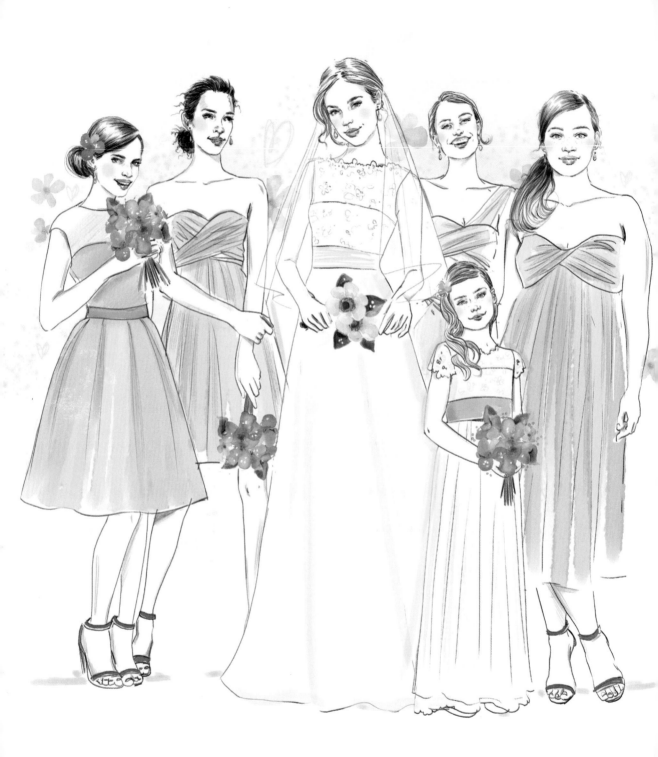

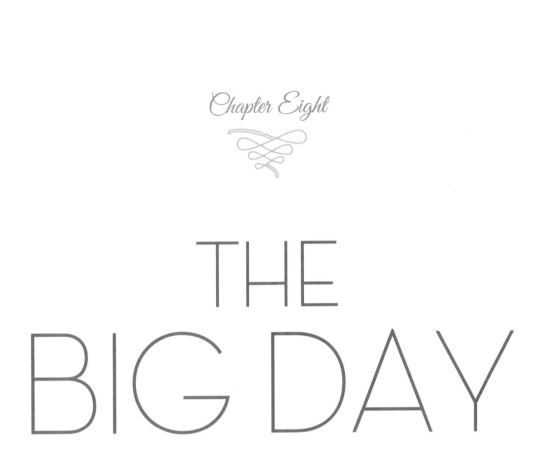

Chapter Eight

THE BIG DAY

YOUR WEDDING DAY IS HERE and you're a mash-up of emotions! Today is all about basking in the enjoyment of it all and embodying your status as the *Radiant Bride*. This is everything you need to know to get you through the hours leading up to saying "I do."

Wake Up to Wed: Your Morning Routine

Depending on the timing of your wedding, the size of your wedding party, and your personal preferences, you'll want to adjust this to fit your schedule. Regardless, don't wait until mere hours before your walk down the aisle to start getting ready. Instead, plan on spending the day with your attendants and taking your time. Enjoy the day. Don't rush. Relax. Relish. Radiate.

GET YOUR Z'S

Nothing is more important the night before your wedding than hitting the hay. Even if you're so excited or nervous that you can't sleep, turn off the lights, close your eyes, and just relax. The restorative rest (even if you never bank a single REM cycle) will give you both the energy you need to feel your best and the rejuvenation you need to look your best.

TAKE YOUR TIME GETTING UP

Your instinct will probably be to pop out of bed. Don't. Spend just a few minutes in bed visualizing the day ahead, taking deep breaths, and relishing the moment. Don't run through to-do lists. Don't stress about what-ifs. Just be in the moment.

CAFFEINATE CAUTIOUSLY

If a cup of Joe is part of your normal morning routine, then by all means go for it. Just be careful not to overdo it. Nothing's worse than a bride with the caffeine jitters! Plus, the adrenaline pumping through your body will likely be all the energy-boosting you need!

EAT

Today is not the day to fast! Nor is it the day to try anything new. Eat breakfast, snack regularly, and make sure to eat right before you put on your dress.

DRINK LOTS OF WATER

I know I'm starting to sound like a broken record but I cannot say it enough! Nothing will ensure your energy levels stay high and your skin shines (in a radiant—not greasy!—way) more than making sure you're not dehydrated.

MOVE

If you have time for a morning spin class or some yoga, go for it! But even if all you have time for is a twenty-minute stroll, having a bit of time to get centered and feel at ease in your body will set the tone for the rest of the day.

SHOWER

You'll feel so refreshed! (Use a shower cap if your hairstylist requested second-day hair, which holds its style a bit more easily!)

EXFOLIATE

In the shower, exfoliate from head to toe to reveal your most radiant complexion. Staying at a hotel? Ask room service for some white sugar packets and mix them with your facial cleanser and/or body wash for a quick and easy scrub on the go.

START WITH A CLEAN SLATE

Discuss with whomever is doing your hair and makeup how they'd like you to start. For most, this will mean a clean face (skincare products you always wear are usually okay, but don't apply any makeup) and day-old hair (meaning you washed it yesterday). But always make sure to ask your stylists.

APPLY SKINCARE

Unless your makeup artist requests otherwise, apply all your usual serums, face creams, eye creams, etc., with ample time for them to soak in before you apply makeup.

WEAR WHITE

Wear a white button-up dress shirt or white bathrobe to get ready in. It will be easier to tell how your makeup will look once you're in your gown if you're wearing a shirt in a similar shade—and avoiding a shirt you have to pull over your head will prevent messing up your hair and makeup.

SEND YOUR GROOM A GIFT

It can be anything from a batch of his favorite cookies to new cufflinks. The price doesn't matter nearly as much as the thought—and the nice note you'll attach! If you're staying at or getting ready in a hotel, the concierge should be able to arrange this for you with enough notice. If not, ask one of your bridesmaids to bring it to wherever he's getting dressed.

THANK EVERYONE
(ESPECIALLY YOUR PARENTS!)

Before the day gets ahead of you, make sure you thank all the people that are making this day so special. Handwritten thank-you notes or a quick toast (with water!) in the bridal suite all work well—and are much appreciated.

MAKEUP

If you're having your makeup professionally done, schedule to do your makeup as early as possible, leaving time for touch-ups right before you walk down the aisle. If you're offering makeup for your bridesmaids, you should go first so pictures of the prep process have your makeup already done. (This is true whether you're having the photographer come by the bridal suite to have in-progress shots taken—which I highly recommend—or just DIYing your wedding prep pictures.) If you're making a schedule for the makeup artist (which you should!), plan for sixty to seventy-five minutes for you and forty-five minutes for each of your bridesmaids, and make sure your makeup artist knows the time constraints and how many girls she'll be responsible for.

HAIR

For your hair, plan on spending sixty minutes (longer if your hair is especially thick or you plan on starting with wet hair). If the women in your wedding party are having their hair done, too, schedule yours for last (just be sure to leave *plenty* of room for makeup touch-ups and getting dressed). If you're traveling to and from a salon (instead of having hairstylists and makeup artists come to your venue), be sure to plan for double the expected time to travel there and back.

MAKE SURE EVERYONE ELSE IS READY

All the women in your wedding party should be ready before you start to get dressed.

SNACK

Before you put on your dress, have a snack. You don't want to risk a spill on your gown (or, for that matter, passing out!).

BODY BEAUTIFYING

Swipe on deodorant (and let it dry!), spray perfume (away from your dress!), and apply body lotion (a kind you've used before and know dries grease-free). If you plan on applying any colored body makeup (like bronzer to your chest), do it now and then buff it in so there isn't any residue. You don't want to get any oils, creams, or sprays on or near your dress so make sure to do *all of this* well before putting on that dress.

GET DRESSED

The moment you've been waiting for: donning that epic gown. Make sure your photographer is there to capture this and to get pictures of your dress before you put it on, too.

ACCESSORIZE

From shoes to jewels, accessorize your look once dressed for gorgeous in-progress photographs. Just make sure to break in those shoes ahead of time. You don't want blisters getting in the way!

ATTACH THE VEIL

If you're wearing a veil, have your hairstylist secure it right before leaving the suite. If you're having your hair done at a salon, have your stylist show your maid of honor how to attach and remove it without messing up your style. If you have the budget for it, have your hairstylist and makeup artist stay until the start of the reception for any touch-ups needed after teary vows—and after removing the veil.

DO A FINAL CHECK

Have your hairstylist and makeup artist give everyone a once-over to make sure everyone is happy. If your makeup artist is leaving, make sure you give your maid of honor any key products for touch-ups, especially lip gloss.

PRECEREMONY PHOTOGRAPHS

If you're doing a "first look," where you see your fiancé for the first time before the ceremony, plan fifteen to twenty minutes for the photographer to capture the moment before having your families arrive, followed by your wedding party. If you're not seeing each other until you walk down the aisle, have the photographer shoot your fiancé, the groomsmen, and your future in-laws together while you finish hair and makeup and then come shoot you, your bridesmaids, and your family. Immediately following the ceremony you can take the remaining photographs. In general, group pictures take two to three minutes each in order to ensure a good shot where all eyes are open and everyone's smiling, so make sure to allot plenty of time. Be sure to discuss this all with your photographer beforehand, in case he or she has other ideas.

PLAN THE ARRIVAL

If you're getting ready somewhere other than where the ceremony will take place, make sure to leave ample time to arrive and have a plan as to where you'll go before walking down the aisle to avoid run-ins with guests before your grand entrance. Take into account your dress's likelihood of wrinkling and consider getting dressed once you arrive.

BREATHE!

Take it all in and enjoy. This is your wedding! You can even ask your officiate to add in a moment of silence so you can take it all in. (He or she doesn't even need to announce it, just ask him or her to pause.)

The Wedding-Day Diet

By this point you know what works for you so eat things you know agree with your body. This isn't the day to try out a new breakfast bar that may or may not sit well in your stomach. Ideally, you'll have quite a few small meals to reduce bloat and keep energy levels consistent, but trust your gut (literally) today.

FIRST THING IN THE MORNING . . .

Eat a breakfast rich in protein and complex carbohydrates. A small bowl of homemade gluten-free granola (turn to page 78 for the recipe) with almond milk, a cup of gluten-free oatmeal topped with raw nuts, or a dairy-free smoothie, are all great choices.

3 HOURS LATER . . .

Refuel with a snack that has fat, protein, and natural sugars to keep you full and satisfied. Try half of an apple with sunflower seed butter, a few stalks of celery with almond butter and raisins, or a cup of carrots with peanut butter. If you're having an evening wedding, this snack should either fall before you even start hair and makeup or in between the two. For a morning wedding, this should take place after your beauty routine is done but before you put on your dress.

LUNCHTIME

Something light but satisfying should make up the bulk of your lunch. This will likely be your last real meal if you're getting married in the evening. A small salad or side of grilled vegetables topped with four ounces of salmon, tofu, or chicken would be ideal. Keep any sauces to a minimum (opting for lemon juice and olive oil instead) to keep thirst and bloat down.

For an evening wedding, this should take place before putting on your dress. For a morning wedding, do your best to find something in this vein at your reception, even if you just take a few bites. This isn't the time to try something you haven't been eating in preparation of this day, though, or you'll run the risk of feeling lethargic and bloated.

AFTERNOON SNACK

For most evening weddings, this will take place between pictures and the ceremony or immediately before pictures. It should be small, but enough to keep your energy high until your wedding is over since you won't likely eat much at the party. It should also be spill-proof! Raw nuts, for example, are a great choice—just ask your maid of honor to feed them to you to avoid getting any oils on your fingers. For most morning weddings, you'll likely skip this snack since you'll be too busy celebrating, but bring it anyway so you can grab a quick bite in the bridal suite, if you remember.

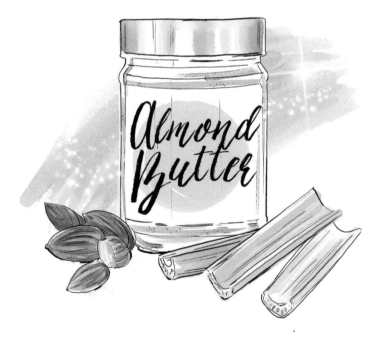

EVENING

No matter the timing of your wedding, you will likely be starving by the end. In fact, most couples say the first thing they do when they get to their bridal suite is . . . wait for it . . . order room service! Since you probably won't have the time (or desire) to sit down and enjoy a meal during your wedding, ask the caterers beforehand to pack up to-go boxes for you and your groom so you can enjoy the leftovers you probably didn't have a chance to enjoy at the reception!

LATE NIGHT

In your overnight bag, pack some healthy, non-perishable snacks and rehydrating beverages so they're there for you if you need them when you finally make it up to the bridal suite.

THROUGHOUT THE DAY

Make sure you're drinking enough fluids! Green juice, coconut water, and water are all great choices! And, as always, listen to your body. Feeling a sugar craving? Listen and respond with fresh fruit or raw chocolate. Pining for salt? Toss raw almonds with a few drops of olive oil and pink sea salt. Your body knows what it needs best, your number-one job is to pay attention.

How to Kick Nerves in the Butt

Don't worry, everything you're feeling is perfectly normal and manageable. Here's how!

DISTRACT. Lean on you bridal backup team and let them know you need a bit of a distraction. They'll likely be grateful for the opportunity to fill you in on their lives, what with all the wedding-prep chat!

LET IT OUT. Sometimes you just need to get those thoughts racing through your mind out of there. Grab a pen and paper and write them down, or call your most understanding brides-maid and open up about how you're feeling. It's normal to be nervous and anxious so don't be embarrassed about sharing your thoughts. The goal here, though, is to let go of the anxiety by diminishing its power, not to ruminate in it—so make sure whoever you call knows that this is about needing someone to listen, not needing someone to tell you how scary it is.

BREATHE DEEPLY. When we're anxious, we naturally start to take more shallow breaths, which makes our bodies feel even more anxious. The result: a downward spiral of nerves. Nip it in the bud by closing your eyes and breathing slowly. Try to breathe in for the count of five, out for the count of six, and repeat. If you're feeling especially on edge, breathe in for five, hold it for two, try to breathe in just a little bit more, and then slowly let it all out for six.

Wedding-Day Don'ts

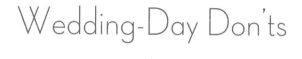

DON'T FORGET TO HAVE FUN. I know you've been dreaming of this day for as long as you can remember (or as long as you've been engaged). And I know you want this day to be "perfect." But remember (for your sake as much as anyone else's), to have fun and let go of the details you can no longer control. No one but you and your wedding planner will notice an off-center floral arrangement.

DON'T FORGET (OR FIGHT WITH) YOUR FIANCÉ. Stress levels are running high—on both ends, probably—and you might both be feeling nervous, anxious, and excited. Remember what brought you here and make sure your love knows it, too.

DON'T PICK AT A PIMPLE! I don't care how big it is. Instead, turn to page 116 and try some of the DIY remedies.

DON'T FORGET TO DRINK WATER. Dehydration is a surefire way to both look and feel sallow.

DON'T EAT ANYTHING TOO SALTY. Not only because sodium bloats, but also because it makes you thirsty—and the last thing you want is to be parched all night long!

DON'T DRINK RED WINE (OR EAT DARK BERRIES). Not just because you most definitely don't want to risk staining your dress, but because they leave a film of darkness on your teeth that will definitely show in pictures.

DON'T FORGET TO SHOW GRATITUDE. For your parents, your bridesmaids, and anyone and everyone who has given you their time or money to make this day as special as possible for you—and that's probably everyone at the wedding.

DON'T SMOKE. You'll be cozied up next to all your nearest and dearest, meeting some of your fiancé's family or friends for the first time, and kissing all night long. You don't want to smell of smoke.

DON'T TAKE DRUGS YOU DON'T NORMALLY TAKE. The day of your wedding is all about being consistent and sticking with what works. In much the way you don't want to try a new exotic fruit juice that may leave you with a stomachache, you don't want to take any drugs (prescription or not) that you don't usually take to avoid risking an adverse reaction. The only exception being if under the care of a doctor, of course.

DON'T DRINK TOO MUCH. This day is going to fly by more quickly than you can possibly imagine. You want to enjoy—and remember—every last bit of it, don't you?!

DON'T FORGET WHAT THIS IS REALLY ALL ABOUT. It's about a marriage, not a wedding, so let love rule the day.

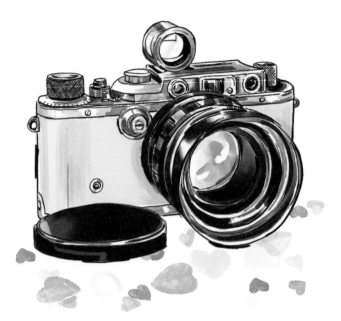

Picture Perfect:
How to Pose for Gorgeous Photos

◇

FIND YOUR BEST SIDE

No one's face is perfectly symmetrical and while I'm sure both sides of your face are gorgeous, you probably have one you like a bit better (even if you don't yet know it!). Take some selfies (or ask your BFF to help you out) and practice posing with your face tilted in each direction. Once you know your "best side," always pose to put your best face forward.

CONTOUR YOUR FACE

A great picture is all about the angles—and a picture taken with you looking directly into the camera flattens out your natural ones by eliminating the shadows that help to contour your face. While that's not to say you can't look stunning in a straight-on shot, if you don't have exceptionally pronounced bone structure, a slight tilt of your chin (either up or down) and turn of your cheek (to your best side, of course) will help to make your face look more chiseled.

MIND YOUR CHIN

To make a round or oval face look slimmer, angle your chin down ever so slightly (careful not to create a double chin in the process!). If you have a pronounced forehead, lift your chin up just a bit to create more balance. Regardless of your face shape and chin angle, push your entire face forward a little. What's closest to the camera will look the biggest, so pushing your face forward a bit will make your body appear slimmer. Alternatively, you can ask the photographer to shoot you from a slightly overhead angle to create the angles without your having to do anything.

SMILE NATURALLY

The key is to smile like you do in real life—and not as big as possible. When you smile largely, your cheeks puff out and your eyes squint, which isn't the most flattering of poses. Instead, practice relaxing your face, opening your mouth ever so slightly, and thinking of something that makes you happy (i.e. spending the rest of your life with your significant other).

USE YOUR TONGUE

Try pushing your tongue up against the roof of your mouth. This somewhat awkward feeling pose will help to elongate your neck and reduce the appearance of any double chin. Just practice ahead of time to make sure you don't look uncomfortable doing it. Apparently models like Heidi Klum do this, and she's not paid the big bucks for nothing!

SMIZE

Tyra Banks popularized the term as shorthand for smiling with your eyes—and it works! You know when you smile how your eyes squint, the corners turn up, and you look slightly up? When you pose, try to replicate that look, even in non-smiling shots. The result will be a more approachable, happy look, even when you're not actually smiling.

ACCENTUATE YOUR ARMS

The key to posing your arms is to keep them away from your body so they're not smushed against your torso, causing them to photograph wider than they actually are. One of the most flattering poses is to put the arm closest to the camera on your hip to accentuate your waist and slim your arm (just be sure to tuck your elbow so it's pointing behind you and not out to the side). Feeling too posed? Just make sure your arms are lifted ever so slightly off your body or hold the person's back next to you to conceal your arm altogether.

LOVE YOUR LEGS

Even if you're wearing a gown that completely conceals your legs, don't forget to pay attention to your legs. Either bend one knee (even the littlest bit) so you don't look stiff or cross your ankles at your calves to elongate your legs and make your hips appear narrower.

ANGLE YOUR BODY

Turn your body so it's at a 45-degree angle or so you're facing the person you are standing next to in order to put your body's depth (not width) on display, which, for most women, is more flattering.

STAND UP STRAIGHT

Great posture goes a long way in making you look happier, healthier, more fit, and more confident. It also affects how you feel: giving you more energy, which you'll need!

RELAX

Have fun, laugh, and be you. You want your pictures to capture the essence of the occasion, not to look posed. Feeling stuck and uptight with all eyes on you? Look away from the camera, or have a moment with your love, and then come back to it. Or when all else fails, dance around a bit!

DON'T FORGET . . .

- **TO HAVE YOUR MAID OF HONOR OR WEDDING PLANNER GATHER MEMENTOS FROM THE PARTY.** *You'll likely be too busy to do it yourself, but you'll be grateful to have a cocktail napkin with your monogram, the place setting card with your names on it, and any other personalized trinkets.*

- **TO ASK EVERYONE TO SEND YOU THE PICTURES THEY TOOK.** *These days everyone has a digital camera. Pre-write an e-mail you can send the morning after (or you can ask your maid of honor to send), asking all of your guests to forward you their pictures. Worried about it clogging your inbox? Create a new e-mail address just for this!*

- **TO BRING YOUR OVERNIGHT BAG.**

- **TO BRING YOUR BRIDAL SURVIVAL KIT** *(see next chapter for everything you need).*

- **THAT EVERYTHING WILL BE OKAY**—*better than okay!—even if your future mother-in-law is running a few minutes late, or the caterer serves red peppers instead of yellow.*

- **TO EAT.** *Okay, I've said this already, but I can't emphasize it enough. Just look on YouTube and you'll see a slew of fainting brides. We don't want you to be one of them!*

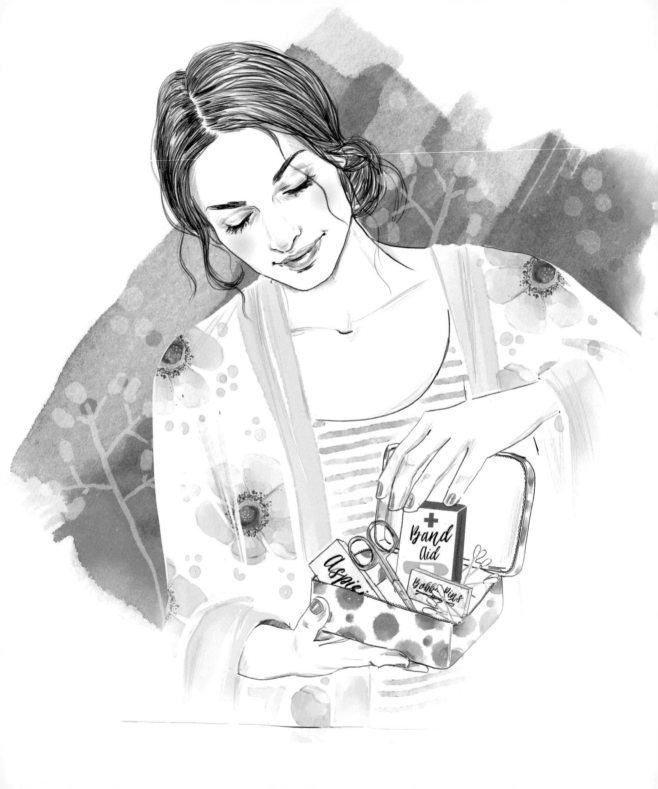

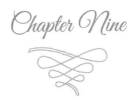

Chapter Nine

BRIDAL 911: YOUR DAY-OF SURVIVAL GUIDE

YOU THINK YOU HAVE EVERYTHING PLANNED BUT, nevertheless, sometimes things go awry. Through the tips in this chapter, you'll be prepared for anything and everything so a torn hemline or giant pimple doesn't ruin your big day.

Packing the Perfect Bridal Survival Kit

The key to a flawless wedding isn't avoiding disaster; it's being prepared. More specifically, it's about preparing for the worst (and, of course, hoping for the best!) with a bridal survival kit. This is the kind of stuff every celebrity stylist has on hand at photo shoots, red carpets, and yes, at celebrity weddings, to ensure all the what-ifs are taken care of!

Having quick and easy access to all of your "in case of emergency" products is just as important as actually having them, so organization is key. To get started, you'll need a large cosmetics bag. My top pick is the kind with lots of clear, plastic, smaller bags nestled within, which you can find at most beauty supply shops—although lots of small plastic Ziploc bags will do the trick as well. Another option is the kind of toiletry organizer you can hang either over the door or on the doorknob of the bathroom. Just make sure you have it in your bridal suite and that you put one of your bridesmaids in charge of bringing it to the wedding reception venue.

THE MUSTS

MAKEUP: Depending on your skin and the makeup you're wearing, this will differ for everyone, but some powder, concealer, and lip gloss are definite must-haves. Ask your makeup artist if he or she has any other suggestions.

OIL BLOTTING SHEETS: Unlike powder that can look ashy when applied too many times throughout the night, these convenient sheets actually absorb the oil instead of merely covering it up—and without messing up your makeup.

Q-TIPS + MAKEUP REMOVER: In the event unexpected tears creep up during the ceremony, you'll be glad to have some clean-up tools!

DEODORANT: For touch-ups—or in case someone in your bridal party forgets. Just make sure it's a clear dry formula.

DEODORANT-REMOVING SPONGE: Have a bridesmaid who failed to jump on the clear deodorant bandwagon? Wipe away the evidence with a sponge designed to remove deodorant sans water.

DOUBLE-SIDED FASHION TAPE: From a spaghetti strap that keeps slipping to a hemline that's come undone, stick fabric to itself—or skin—with this multi-use, fashionista must-have.

SEWING KIT + SAFETY PINS: You never know when a good old needle and thread will come in handy—or when you'll need safety pins to secure a broken dress strap or remove a splinter. If possible, ask your wedding dress designer (or the salesperson) if they have a swatch of the thread used on your gown in case you need it to reattach a strap or otherwise troubleshoot).

HAIR TIES + BOBBY PINS: You got your hair done for the big day but dancing's left it messy? You'll be grateful for your ability to fix it on the fly (or for your maid of honor to do it!).

HAIR SPRAY: Sure, it tames frizzy flyaways and secures falling up-dos, but did you know it can also remove lipstick stains from your man's shirt?

STATIC GUARD: While hair spray can sometimes do the trick, don't risk ruining fabrics with this made-for-clothes static solution.

LINT-REMOVING ROLL: Because you may love your pet, but you don't love their hair making a cameo in all your pictures.

STAIN-REMOVING STICK OR WIPE: It's like an insurance policy: you hope you don't need it, but you sure are glad you have it on hand if you do.

NAIL FILE: Snag a nail? Instead of picking at it all night (like I would!) or scratching yourself (or others) repeatedly, fix it pronto.

BAND-AIDS: Cuts, blisters, hangnails, oh my! Just make sure they're clear so they're invisible on all skin tones.

ANTIHISTAMINES: Runny noses and watery eyes are never a good thing. Hives are even worse. Treat all of the above with an over-the-counter antihistamine.

ASPIRIN: It's not just for when your future mother-in-law comes down with a migraine, but also for reducing the appearance of a pimple, too! Just crush one aspirin in a few drops of water and apply to the spot for a couple of minutes. Rinse off and conceal with makeup!

ANTACIDS: Just in case nerves give you a sour stomach—or the best man eats one too many passed hors d'oeuvres.

CORTISONE CREAM: On bug bites, rashes, and other irritations, it will help to assuage discomfort and reduce redness.

BREATH MINTS + TOOTHPICKS: You'll be close-talking with all your friends and family over the music—and kissing your newly betrothed all night. Make sure your breath is minty fresh and there's no food in your teeth. Look for breath mints at a health food store that are made without any artificial sweeteners, which can upset your stomach.

TOOTHBRUSH + PASTE: You'll want one last brush after you eat your final pre-gown meal and before you apply your lipstick.

TISSUES: For tears and sniffles—as well as post-kiss lipstick on cheeks.

TAMPONS: You never know how stressors like a wedding can affect your cycle—or if someone in your wedding party will have forgotten her own.

SHOE PADS + MOLESKIN: If your feet start to ache or your shoes start to slip, you'll be thankful you have them.

ANTI-REDNESS EYEDROPS: They're great post-tears (and post-hangover!).

SUPERGLUE: To reattach a heel on a shoe or beads on a dress.

SMALL SCISSORS: Just in case.

WHITE CHALK: Cover up a stain on your dress with white chalk if you're in a bind.

COMFORTABLE SHOES: Whether flip-flops or sneakers, bring an extra pair of shoes so you can dance the night away sans heels (and blisters)!

GREAT ATTITUDE: It's not a matter of if something will go "wrong," it's a matter of what it will be and when. Nothing, though, should get in the way of your ability to enjoy your big day. Sure, a big red wine stain on your gown isn't ideal, but would you rather spend your wedding in the bathroom crying about it, or enjoying the party you've spent months planning anyway? Today is about celebrating your love and your commitment to spend the rest of your lives together, the rest is just icing on the cake. (Sometimes literally.)

THE MAYBE-HAVES

DRY SHAMPOO: If you're wearing your hair down and it's prone to falling flat, use dry shampoo to give it a volumizing boost. Just make sure it's a formula that either matches the color of your hair or dries invisibly. We aren't going for a powdered Marie Antoinette look.

PERFUME: Toss your favorite perfume in your kit if you want to touch up your fragrance during the evening. Just make sure to use a solid or rollerball—not a spray, which can stain your dress! And remember that your nose becomes desensitized, so make sure you're not applying too much.

MATTIFYING POWDER: If your skin is oily and prone to breakthrough shine, keep a translucent mattifying powder on hand to control shine without messing up your makeup.

BABY POWDER: Worried about sweaty, sticky, swollen feet? A dash of baby powder in your shoes will help!

STRAWS: Wearing a dramatic lipstick or high-shine gloss? Sip your drinks without leaving most of your lip color behind by using a straw. You'll also be less likely to inadvertently spill your drink on your dress. Just be sure to sip slowly to try to minimize the amount of air you swallow, which can lead to bloating.

BLISTER BLOCKERS: Whether you prefer a blister-blocking stick or gel insoles, plan for the worst-case scenario with a blister-blocking solution that fits in your shoes.

EXTRA HOSIERY: If you're wearing hose, make sure you have a backup pair on hand!

EXTRA SOCKS: For him.

EXTRA DRESS SHIRT: For him, in case he sweats or spills—or gets your makeup on his shirt.

NAIL POLISH: If a small chip will drive you crazy, bring the exact shade with you for a touch-up on the go.

NAIL POLISH REMOVER: If you're wearing a darker shade than nude, bring nail polish remover just in case. Just be sure it's securely stored to avoid a second beauty disaster!

CROCHET HOOK: If your dress—or your attendants' dresses—have buttons with loop closures, this will help ease the process.

UMBRELLA: If your wedding venue poses any risk of rain—and of subjecting you to it—it's better to be safe than sorry!

FULL-FAT GREEK YOGURT: It's one of my favorite facial masks and an amazing spot treatment for immediately reducing the appearance of any facial redness or even a pimple. Just make sure you have a refrigerator to store it in!

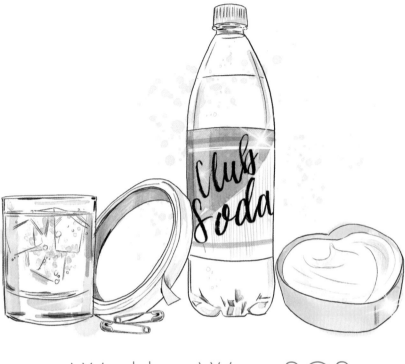

Wedding Woes SOS

IF YOU SPILL ON YOUR DRESS . . .

The key to cleaning up a spill is to dab, not rub—and to do so ASAP. Use a cloth damped with water or club soda and dab the spot until no more of the stain is coming up. Then, let it dry before covering up with white chalk. Take the dress to an experienced dry cleaner immediately after the wedding (or ask your maid of honor to do so if you're off on your honeymoon).

IF YOU HAVE PUFFY EYES . . .

Spent all night up with your girlfriends or the morning crying with your mom? Cure puffy eyes easily at an event venue. Just ask for a cup of ice water and two metal spoons. Soak the spoons in the water to chill before applying on your eyes (with the back on the spoons gently pressing in your eye socket) for a few minutes. Repeat as needed.

IF YOUR DRESS BREAKS . . .

If your hem comes undone from dancing, have your bridesmaids help you to secure it using the double-sided tape and/or safety pins in your emergency kit. If the strap snaps, use the sewing kit, if possible, or a safety pin.

IF YOUR MASCARA RUNS . . .

Use a Q-tip and some makeup remover (or even some Vaseline or coconut oil!) to carefully remove running makeup. Dab dry before reapplying makeup, as needed.

YOU GET A GIANT ZIT . . .

Stress is a major skin aggravator so it's not unusual to break out on the big day. Rule #1: DON'T PICK IT! The best option is to call your dermatologist and have it injected with cortisone to immediately reduce the puffiness and redness.

Not an option? Apply a small dab of full-fat Greek yogurt and let it sit for fifteen minutes (or longer). The lactic acid helps to break down the clogged pore and reduce redness and puffiness, the probiotics balance bacteria, and the fat moisturizes for a surface perfectly primed for makeup.

No yogurt to be found? Head to your emergency kit and get crafty. Start by crushing an aspirin in a few drops of water to create a paste. Apply that to the pimple for a few minutes (remove it immediately if you feel any irritation) before rinsing off. Then saturate a Q-tip with the anti-redness eyedrops and hold it on the pimple for a few minutes. Finally, conceal it!

IF YOUR SHOE BREAKS . . .

Walking down the aisle should be one of the best moments of your life, not ripe with anxiety. Scuff your shoes on a driveway or sidewalk before the wedding so they're not slippery and walk around in them for a couple of days to get your footing. And, in the off chance your heel breaks, either ditch your shoes and put on the comfortable pair you (should have) brought with you, or reattach the heel with the superglue in your emergency kit.

IF YOUR NAIL POLISH CHIPS . . .

Use your nail file to gently buff any rough edges before applying a fresh coat of polish to the entire nail. Just make sure to do this far away from your dress!

IF A GROOMSMAN FORGETS HIS TIE . . .

Have your wedding planner (or best man) call a local rental store and see if they can messenger one over. Otherwise, talk with the photographer. He or she can likely position the forgetful fellow so as to minimize attention. Alternatively, you can ask all groomsmen to ditch the tie if your wedding's dress code allows.

IF YOUR ENGAGEMENT RING IS STUCK . . .

Whether you plan on wearing your wedding and engagement rings stacked or on separate hands, prior to your ceremony you'll want to move your engagement ring to your right hand to make putting your wedding band on easier.

Fingers swollen from traveling or climate change and it won't budge? Don't panic. Submerge your hand in ice water to reduce swelling before applying hand lotion, oil, or hair conditioner to your finger and wiggling the ring off. Just make sure you don't do this over the sink or near any drain! Reapply a bit of lotion, oil, or hair conditioner before walking down the aisle, too, so it's easier to slip on your wedding band during the ceremony.

IF YOU HAVE A HANGOVER . . .

Treat it like you would any other hangover (and head back to Chapter 4 for a refresher course).

IF YOU'RE DEALING WITH BUG BITES . . .

Whether the itchiness or unsightliness is the biggest concern, apply a cortisone cream to the affected areas to reduce redness, inflammation, and discomfort. If it's really unbearable, consider taking one of the antihistamines in your emergency kit, just be careful because they can make you groggy.

IF YOU'RE FEELING ANXIOUS . . .

Your walk down the aisle should be dramatic, but not because you're having a panic attack! If you're feeling anxious, surround yourself with calming love and avoid any heart-racing beverages like coffee, caffeinated soda, and energy drinks. Some brides find that seeing their soon-to-be-betrothed eases nerves, so if the anxiety becomes too much, consider breaking your ban on seeing each other before the ceremony so you can calm down and enjoy the wedding.

IF YOU GET MAKEUP ON YOUR GROOM'S SHIRT . . .

Ask someone in your bridal party to help you to use the stain-removing sticks or wipes in your bridal survival kit to clean his shirt while he changes into the spare. Hang the dirty shirt, though, so in the event the second one is spilled on, the first one isn't a wrinkled mess.

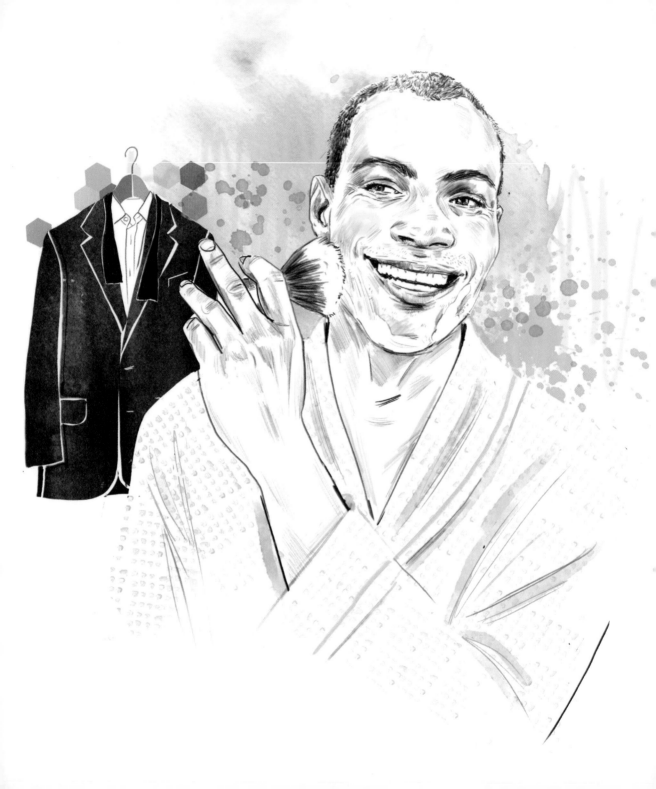

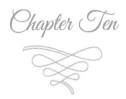

Chapter Ten

GETTING GROOMED

YOUR MAN MAY NOT THINK HE NEEDS TO PREP for the big day, but we both know better! From when to get his hair cut to how to calm razor burn stat, this chapter will give you the tools you need to ensure he looks as handsome as you do beautiful on the big day. Either pass this chapter on to him or just gently suggest he follow the below—you'll both appreciate the results!

Whether your man is a face-wash novice or manscaping connoisseur, getting him to jump on an entirely new beauty regimen may be a challenge. And, thankfully, it's not required.

Fact is: you fell in love with him regardless of his grooming habits (as he did with you), so now's not the time to be nitpicking the particulars of his routine. So, you ask, what's the point of this section? It's for the man who has either been raiding your beauty supplies in an attempt to subtly tap into his inner beauty king, the entirely clueless gent who's looking for some direction, or the man for whom whatever he's currently doing just isn't working. Also, it's for the man who couldn't care less about any of this, until, that is, he wakes up the morning of the big day with a photographer *en route* and a pimple smack dab in the middle of his forehead. No matter where he falls on the spectrum, however, just make sure he doesn't try anything new within two weeks of your wedding to avoid any potential adverse reactions.

Think of this as the CliffsNotes version of Chapter 6 designed for you—although, by all means, if your man is up for it, put him on the more elaborate beauty prescription outlined in Chapter 6!

Grooming the Groom's Hair (Everywhere!)

HEAD HAIR

Most men, like women, know that they're happiest with their hair a few days (sometimes longer) after a cut. Start paying attention now to when he likes his post-cut 'do best and make sure he schedules his pre-wedding cut at the right time so it's perfect for the big day. This would also be a good time to ensure he has a regular go-to person for his haircut (and not just a go-to place) who is familiar with just how he likes it. You definitely don't want to start experimenting with a new style or a new pair of scissor-bearing hands before this momentous (and widely photographed!) day.

FACIAL HAIR

Unless you're a stellar shaver (and I mean, award-winning), you should avoid taking blade to skin on the big day lest any unforeseen cut or irritation occur. Want a clean-shaven look? Shave the night before and use an electric razor to touch-up the morning of. A little stubble is better than an unexpected cut or razor burn.

BODY HAIR

So, this is the stuff most men (and women) don't want to talk about, but here we go anyway. While "manscaping" has become exponentially more popular over the last few decades, in much the same way a Brazilian bikini wax isn't for everyone, body hair removal isn't for every man. Thankfully, unlike your body, his is pretty covered up at all but the most unconventional of weddings. That being said, if you're having a destination wedding where you'll be lounging beachside pre- and post-nuptials, consider your hair removal options.

EYEBROWS

Many men think brow grooming is just for the ladies, but those men are wrong. Few celebrity men I know don't at least clean up the area between their brows to fix a potential unibrow! While I'd advise a visit to a brow expert (especially one used to working with men since the last thing you want are too-tamed, ladylike brows), if that's too much to ask of your man, carefully help your fiancé to tweeze the hairs between his brows and subtly trim long brow hairs, if needed.

Lucky enough to have a man willing to trust the pros? Schedule his first visit at least three months before to ensure he doesn't have an adverse reaction to the process—or the result! Schedule his pre-wedding appointment when you do your own (two weeks before the big day). And never—I repeat: never!—shave between the brows.

NOSE + EAR HAIR

Few things are as unsexy as nose and ear hair. Not all men have it, but those that do far too often are blissfully unaware. While pointing out a partner's flaws is never a good thing, if your man has some unnoticed strays in his nose or ears, considering buying him a trimmer made just for that purpose and gently encouraging him to use it. Don't ever use tweezers or regular scissors, though, as they can seriously injure both sensitive areas.

Hair Removal 101

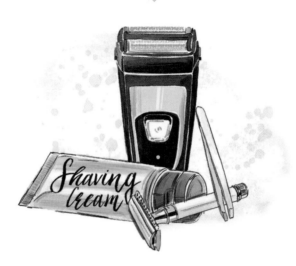

RAZOR

PROS:	Very affordable. A razor gives a super-close shave.
CONS:	It can leave you with razor burn and ingrown hairs, especially on never-before-shaved areas, and cuts are always a risk, even for pro-shavers.
TIPS:	Exfoliate beforehand for a closer shave, and don't do it right before the wedding in case you cut yourself.
BEST FOR:	The back of the neck and facial hair

ELECTRIC RAZOR

PROS:	Very low risk of razor burn or ingrown hairs. You can use it the day of the big event, easy to DIY.
CONS:	Not as close of a shave as a traditional razor (a larger con for men with thick, coarse hair)
TIPS:	Make sure the razor's cutter is clean and start on the most sensitive areas, working toward less sensitive areas (since the razor can get warm during use, causing irritation). Exfoliate beforehand for a closer shave.
BEST FOR:	When you want to leave a bit (or a lot) of scruff or just clean up a beard, day-of touch-ups, sideburns, and below-the-belt (aka pubic) manscaping

TWEEZING

PROS:	Extremely precise, very low risk of irritation at the time of removal (so long as you don't accidently nab your skin). Tweezing removes hair from the root so the results last longer.
CONS:	Time-consuming and can be painful, can increase risk of ingrown hairs for people prone to them
TIPS:	Apply warm compresses to the area for a few minutes prior to tweezing to open the pores, for easier removal.
BEST FOR:	Areas with few hairs to remove and/or when precision is key

DEPILATORY CREAM

PROS:	Quick and painless
CONS:	It can irritate even not-so-sensitive skin (so definitely do a spot test well before the big day!) and hair grows back as quickly as with shaving.
TIPS:	Make sure you test this on a small, hidden area and then wait twenty-four hours to make sure no reaction occurs before using this on a larger area.
BEST FOR:	Men who are pain averse and/or have a large amount of body hair to remove

WAX

PROS:	Great for removing large areas of hair. The results last up to three weeks, and the hair grows in softer than with shaving.
CONS:	Painful, expensive at a salon, and difficult to DIY. Wax can cause burns, irritation, and ingrown hairs.
TIPS:	Exfoliate beforehand to ensure all hairs are primed for removal. Make sure skin is clean and lotion-free before waxing. Apply an over-the-counter cortisone cream to waxed areas to reduce irritation.
BEST FOR:	Large areas like the back and shoulders

ELECTROLYSIS

PROS:	Permanent
CONS:	Expensive, very time-consuming (since each hair needs to be individually treated)
TIPS:	Make sure you're not a candidate for laser hair removal first.
BEST FOR:	People with light hair or dark skin (since lasers work best when there is contrast between hair and skin color) who are looking for a permanent solution

LASER HAIR REMOVAL

PROS:	Permanent
CONS:	Expensive, requires multiple sessions (although it's far less time-consuming than electrolysis if you're treating a large area). Most important: if it's not done by a trained professional, it can cause permanent scarring to your skin.
TIPS:	Make sure you go to a dermatologist or a highly qualified technician specifically trained in and certified to perform laser hair removal. Also, if you're treating a very sensitive area, ask for numbing cream.
BEST FOR:	People with dark hair and light skin since the laser works by targeting contrast

Razor Burn + Ingrown Hairs SOS

RAZOR BURN

Even the most practiced of hair removing gents sometimes hit a snag. Whether it's a new razor that's tripped you up or skin that's more sensitive from climate changes, calm the irritation with this remedy:

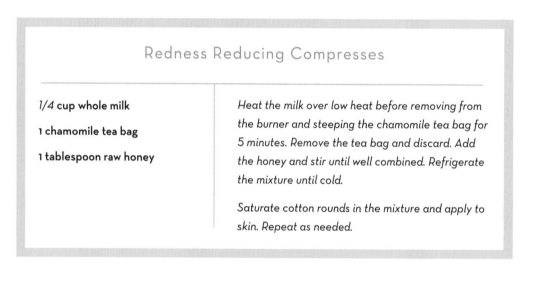

Redness Reducing Compresses

1/4 cup whole milk	Heat the milk over low heat before removing from the burner and steeping the chamomile tea bag for 5 minutes. Remove the tea bag and discard. Add the honey and stir until well combined. Refrigerate the mixture until cold.
1 chamomile tea bag	
1 tablespoon raw honey	
	Saturate cotton rounds in the mixture and apply to skin. Repeat as needed.

Quick Tip

Save chill time by adding ice cubes once the mixture is cooled to room temperature.

INGROWN HAIRS

If you're a chronic sufferer, start experimenting with new hair removal techniques well before the wedding date in order to find the one best suited for your skin and hair. It's also time you start a prophylactic routine. The key: exfoliation to prevent hairs trying to grow in from getting trapped underneath dead skin cells. Whether you prefer a chemical exfoliant (like an astringent or saturated cleansing pad packed with skin-rejuvenating acids that you can find at your local drugstore, spa, or barbershop) or a manual exfoliator (like a grainy body scrub or just a handful of white sugar), removing the dead skin cells every couple of days will keep your skin clear and ingrown hairs at bay.

While prevention is the best medicine, if you find yourself in a bind with a last-minute ingrown hair, it isn't anything to fret over. Instead, try making this:

Skin-Soothing Spot Treatment

| 1 teaspoon full-fat Greek yogurt | Mix both ingredients together until smooth. Apply a thin layer to affected areas and let sit for 15 minutes before rinsing with warm water. |
| 1/2 teaspoon raw honey | |

Quick Tips

While I don't recommend ever trying something new right before saying "I do," if you find yourself with your first ingrown hair on the big day, this spot treatment is pretty safe even for sensitive skin (assuming you're not allergic to any of the ingredients). Just to be safe, though, apply a small dab on the inside of your wrist and let it sit for fifteen minutes to test for a reaction before applying this on your face.

No yogurt or honey in sight? Apply a thick layer of an over-the-counter corti-sone cream to reduce redness. Rinse it off when you need to start getting ready.

Last, but not least, find your bride-to-be's makeup artist and ask for some concealer—there's no shame in a bit of cover-up!

Skincare Saviors:
Daily Solutions + Day-of Savers

◇

DRY SKIN

Try using extra-virgin cold-pressed coconut oil instead of your usual nightly moisturizer. It's packed with fats to hydrate, but what really makes this a dry skin saver is its lauric acid, which helps to gently exfoliate dry, dead skin cells, so the moisturizing properties can really work their magic. Prefer a more traditional lotion? Look for ones that are both alcohol-free and contain hyaluronic acid and/or natural oils (like olive, argan, and coconut). Also, make sure you're exfoliating at least two times per week—and especially the day of—to polish away dull, dry skin.

ACNE

If your skin is constantly breaking out and consistently oily, try adding more anti-inflammatory and rejuvenating foods to your diet (like berries and carrots, respectively) and drinking more water. Cutting out dairy and gluten can also help, so it's at least worth a try. As for skincare, make sure you're not over-drying. As counterintuitive as it may sound, drying out your skin could be the problem. Even if your skin is still appearing oily. When your skin is too dry, it panics and starts to over-compensate by producing sebum (the pore-clogging kind of oil). Keep your skin moisturized (ideally with an anti-inflammatory and antibacterial moisturizer like extra-virgin cold-pressed coconut oil) and your body will know that no sebum is necessary. Skin still shiny (and wish it weren't)? Use an oil-controlling moisturizer (lots of men's skincare brands, like Clinique for Men and Anthony Logistics, make them) and apply a mattifying powder. (Urban Decay's De-Slick Mattifying Powder is great because it's clear, so you won't feel like you're wearing any makeup.)

OCCASIONAL BREAKOUTS

If your skin is less acne prone and more just prone to the once in a while breakout, Murphy's Law says that on this all-eyes-on-you day, you'll find yourself with a face full of zits. If your skin is aggravated by stress (or travel, if you will be traveling for your wedding), start to pre-treat your skin two to three weeks before the big day with the products you would usually only use if you were actively breaking out. You do not want to suddenly start a never-before-tried skincare routine before the big day and risk having an allergic reaction, but pre-treating your skin with your current worst-case scenario arsenal will help to keep any impending pimples away.

DAY-OF PIMPLES

If during the day or two leading up to your wedding you wake to find a single giant zit taking over your face, head to the dermatologist who can quickly inject the pimple with cortisone to immediately reduce inflammation and redness. Dealing with more than one—or can't make it to the doc? Now is not the time to try drying them out (you need a couple of days for that to be an effective strategy) or picking (which is *never* a good strategy). Rather, focus on reducing redness and inflammation. My favorite tip: apply a thin layer of full-fat Greek yogurt as a mask. Within a few minutes, it will reduce redness, irritation, and inflammation. Then ask your bride's makeup artist for a little help (yes, it will come in the form of makeup and no, no one will know!).

BODY BREAKOUTS

You're about to embark on a week with (likely!) more nudity than any other before, so now would be a good time to get those body breakouts under control once and for all. Because your body's skin is less sensitive than that of your face, as a general rule of thumb, any acne product designed for your face is also safe for your body (although the reverse isn't true). So, feel free to use any blemish-busting mask designed for your face to spot-treat any body zits. As for regular maintenance, look for a body wash with salicylic acid and use it in the shower daily. If that's still not cutting it, apply medicated acne pads to affected areas nightly before bed.

UNDER-EYE CIRCLES

Often wake with under-eye darkness or puffiness? Add an eye cream with caffeine to your daily routine—and store it in the fridge. The caffeine helps to constrict the blood vessels and reduce under-eye discoloration while the coolness helps to reduce puffiness. Also, try sleeping on your back with an extra pillow to reduce fluid accumulation in your face and getting at least seven hours of sleep.

Have chronic under-eye circles no matter how much sleep you get? They could be caused by a vitamin K deficiency, so start adding more kale and parsley to your diet!

CUTS + BRUISES

Rule #1: avoid cuts and bruises at all costs in the days leading up to your wedding! Dreaming of a new BMX bike? Now's not the time! It's also not the time to throw any punches or get wasted with your buddies (the bachelor party should have taken place weeks ago). Broken rule #1 and in a bind? Here's what you need to know:

1) Ensure there isn't any serious injury that requires medical attention.

2) Address any bleeding or oozing by cleaning the area thoroughly and covering, as needed.

3) Treat any pain or discomfort with over-the-counter pain medicine (just be sure to ask the pharmacist about interactions with alcohol if you're planning on drinking).

4) Find your bride's makeup artist, a bridesmaid, or your mom and ask for some help concealing the injury.

SUNBURN

If the sun's done more than just kiss you and your skin is closer to red than it is to bronze, head to the kitchen. Saturate a soft washcloth in cold whole milk and let it sit on the burned skin until no longer chilled. Repeat regularly. Also, be sure to drink lots of water (and avoid alcohol) to help your body replenish hydration from the inside out. You can also take an over-the-counter anti-inflammatory to help with pain and swelling.

SWEAT

You've been known to sweat through a shirt even when you're feeling calm, cool, and collected, and, well, your wedding isn't likely to be one of those times. Even the most confident grooms (and brides!) are known to feel a bit of nervous excitement. You likely already know the answer to this, but start paying attention to where you typically sweat the most. We all have our "areas," and some are worse than others (sweaty feet: not too problematic on your wedding day; sweaty chest: exponentially more problematic). Then, start testing new antiperspirants to see which ones work best for you and on various parts of your body (yes, you can apply it to your chest, for example). I like Clinical Strength Certain Dri for big occasions—even though it sometimes irritates my sensitive skin. Not cutting it? Talk with your dermatologist about whether you're a good candidate for prescription antiperspirants or even Botox injections to temporarily stop the sweat. Also, make sure you talk to your tailor about the most breathable fabrics as well as the ones least likely to show sweat stains. Really concerned? Talk both with your wedding planner and venue about cranking up the air-conditioning and buy an extra shirt so you can change, if needed!

TEETH

You're about to take more pictures than probably ever before—ideally smiling! Sure, a professional teeth whitening is great, but it's expensive and time-consuming. Instead, switch your toothpaste to a whitening variety, swap your coffee for iced coffee (drinking from a straw helps bypass your teeth and prevents stains!), and try using Crest 3D White Whitestrips, which can whiten your teeth just as much as a professional treatment for a fraction of the cost (and without having to spend an hour or more in a dentist's office). And for an added DIY bonus, polish your teeth manually by dipping a damp toothbrush in pure baking soda and brushing as usual.

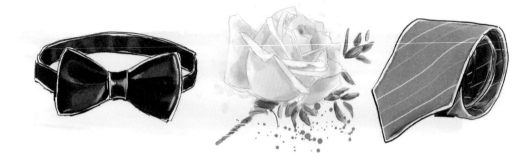

Groom's Garb

I'm going to make this quick since this book is, after all, about the ladies! That being said, when it comes to living happily ever after with wedding pictures you love, having your man dressed for the occasion is likely important to you. So, here's what you both need to know.

Like with the bride's dress, the groom's attire should make him feel like a rock star (ripped jeans and concert tee not suggested). The only true "rule" is that he be dressed no less formally than the dress code called for on the invite. Indicating a black-tie wedding on your invitation? He should be in a tuxedo. That's not to say, though, that you can't dress more formally than you're calling for guests to dress. Specifying cocktail attire on your invite? A suit is the minimal level of formality you should don, but you can always dress more formally and rock a tux.

TUXEDO + SUIT

While a tuxedo is standard for a black-tie wedding, for any other level of formality there is quite a bit of flexibility as to what the groom can and should wear. My one rule of thumb: go for timeless over trendy—and always splurge on an excellent tailor. Colors, cummerbunds, and pleats can date you, but a timeless, well-fitted suit will look fabulous forever.

Before suit shopping, help streamline the process and reduce in-store stress by taking some time beforehand to look through magazines and his closet to get a better idea of each of your preferences. And, as always, know your budget before beginning.

SHIRT

For most grooms, the part of the shirt that matters most, both in terms of comfort and style, is the collar. Before deciding on a shirt, make sure you try on a branded collar (like an ultra-mini mock turtleneck or super-high crew neck, which pairs well with any neckwear); a winged collar (like that on a typical suit's dress shirt, which also pairs well with any neckware); a turndown collar (for use with a bowtie or simple necktie); and a Windsor collar (which spreads out widely to accommodate a tie fashioned with a Windsor knot). Whatever you decide, consider buying a second shirt just in case you spill on it during the cocktail hour.

TIE + BOWTIE

Before you commit to a bowtie, try it on and wear it around the house for a few hours. Most men feel like they're choking, a sensation any man should avoid at all costs on his wedding day! Regardless of whether you choose a bowtie or tie, keep it simple. Considering matching the men's ties or bowties with the bridesmaids' dresses? Just be sure it's classic and subtle (shades of silver or gray are best), and not hot pink.

VEST OR WAISTCOAT

Increasingly popular with a tuxedo or suit—and a decidedly more modern accessory than the cummerbund—the vest can be either single or double breasted, just ensure it matches the jacket. If you're planning on taking off your jacket at any point during the night (and you probably will!), it's worth spending the extra money on a full vest, which has the same fabric on the back as on the front (versus less pricey vests, which cut costs by fashioning the back with an inexpensive fabric but are designed to be worn only when your jacket will remain on all night long).

BOUTONNIERE

It's a great way to tie the wedding party together (especially if all the groomsmen are dressed in simple black), but definitely optional. If you do decide to don a boutonniere, only do so on a jacket with a specific boutonniere buttonhole on the lapel to avoid damaging the fabric of your jacket. And keep it simple to avoid looking like you're off to prom. This is also a great way to differentiate the groom from his groomsmen. Bonus points if it matches the bride's bouquet!

RENTING VS. BUYING

If your man's weight fluctuates, or your next formal affair will be, oh, I don't know, approximately fifteen years from now, you'll want to rent your wedding-day formal wear. Styles (and bodies) change, so if you don't regularly attend formal affairs, renting will be your best choice. If, however, you think you'll use the tux at least three or four times, it's likely worth buying.

Don't forget to have your outfit professionally pressed prior to the wedding to ensure it's perfectly wrinkle-free. If you're having a destination wedding, talk with the accommodations ahead of time to ensure this is something they can take care of in a timely manner.

THE GROOMSMEN

Just as with the bridesmaids' dresses, you want the groomsmen to look cohesive, but that doesn't mean they need to match (the only exception, a very formal/traditional black-tie wedding). For a formal wedding, ask all the groomsmen to wear a black tuxedo, but let them wear one they already own or choose one they find most flattering. Wedding more casual? Ask them all to wear the same colored jacket. Like with sashes on bridesmaid gowns, consider purchasing a unique pocket square, bowtie, or tie to help them all to look both cohesive and stand out.

9 Tips for the Groom (No Peeking, Brides!)

You bought a ring, popped the question, and she said yes! Think your job is done? Think again, sir.

1) APPROACH EVERYTHING WITH LOVE. You may think her fretting over flowers is absurd, but it's in neither of your best interests to tell her that. This is about a marriage, not just a wedding, and if I know anything about what's led to my parents' fifty-plus years of wedded bliss, it's having open ears, minds, and hearts—and approaching everything from a place filled with love.

2) HAVE AN OPINION. This is a celebration of both of you, so make sure your voice is heard. Love food? Take charge of the menu. Dream about being a DJ? Now's your chance! Not only will you feel more included, your bride-to-be will be thrilled you're both taking interest and that you're taking things off her plate!

3) SELECT, MANAGE, + REWARD THE MEN. You're responsible for picking the men who will stand up with you at your wedding. Other than being sure to include your brother(s) and hers (no matter how close—or not close—you are), whom you choose to be a part of your bridal party is entirely up to you. (And, no, you don't need to match the number of bridesmaids she has. Closeness is considerably more important that consistency.)

Once selected, keep your groomsmen in the loop as to pre-nuptial and day-of responsibilities and ensure they are on board. (Have a friend who always loses his phone? Probably not the best man to put in charge of your rings!) Remember, you probably didn't know much about how all this worked before you got engaged, so make sure to give your groomsmen plenty of notice as to exactly what is being asked of them. Will they need to get fitted for a tux? Make sure they know when they need to do it, where to go, and how much it will cost. Also be sure to include the details both for picking up and returning the tux (to avoid late fees). And, finally, don't forget to get your groomsmen a thoughtful thank-you gift.

4) PREPARE A TOAST. If you're having a rehearsal dinner, saying a few words to your bride-to-be and both of your families is a customary (and great!) way to set the celebration off on the right foot. If you're not having a rehearsal dinner, while you're taking photographs would be a great time to express your thanks.

Terrified of speaking in front of crowds? Pull your parents and future in-laws aside and express your gratitude in private. Additionally, handwritten notes to your parents, future in-laws, and bride-to-be will go a long way! At formal weddings, it's also customary to speak at the wedding, but this is less of a steadfast rule, just make sure everyone (who needs to) knows your plan.

5) BE SENTIMENTAL. If you're writing your own vows, get down and dirty with your emotions. If not, send a handwritten note to the room she's getting ready in or leave it on her bed for her to read after the rehearsal dinner.

6) BUY HER A WEDDING GIFT. You may think that you're gift enough (and you are) but that doesn't mean you shouldn't commemorate this day with more than just the most expensive party you've ever thrown. Jewelry is always a safe bet but feel free to get creative. Just ensure it's both personal and memorable—and something she'll have forever.

7) PARTY SMARTLY. There are lots of reasons to celebrate—and lots of occasions to do it—but make sure to do so smartly. Heading off for your bachelor party? Have fun but be respectful of your bride-to-be. Psyched to see your best buds from college at your rehearsal dinner? Now's not the time to go shot-for-shot.

8) EXTRA CREDIT. Surprise her with a massage to taper prewedding stress, send her flowers to let her know how excited you are, or take her out on a romantic date to the place of your first date the week before.

9) TAKE CONTROL OF THE HONEYMOON. No matter how into (or not into) wedding planning you are, everyone enjoys a vacation! Take over the planning of the honeymoon and you'll not only take something off her plate, you'll also be able to plan the trip of your dreams.

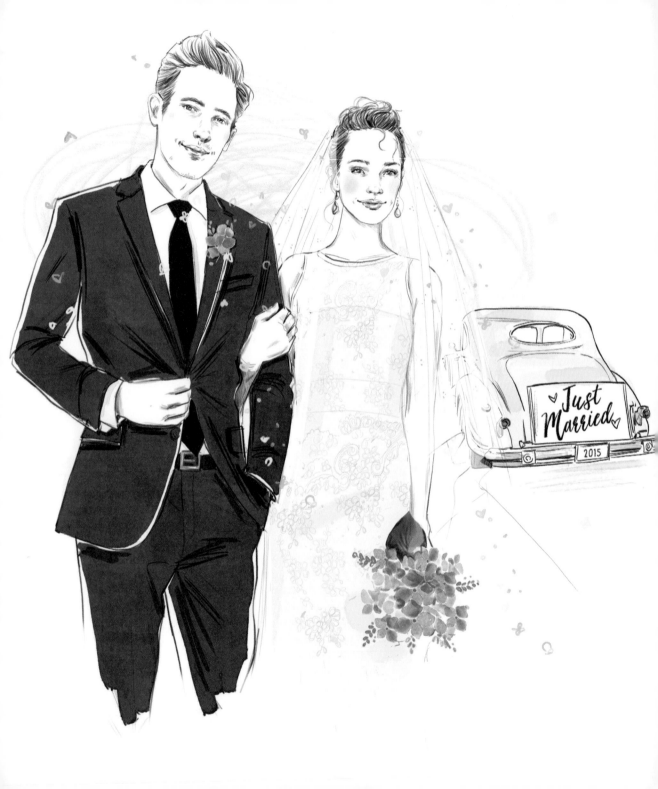

BON VOYAGE!
THE
HONEYMOON

WANT TO LOOK AND FEEL LIKE YOUR SEXIEST SELF?

Well, newsflash: you already do! Love looks good on everyone and you're definitely no exception. Plus, you've been working your butt off to look and feel like your most beautiful self. Now it's time to relish in it all!

By the time everyone wishes you *bon voyage*, your big day may be over, but the real trip is just beginning—and, no, I'm not just talking about your honeymoon. Whether you're hitting the road immediately after your wedding or waiting to take your honeymoon in celebration of your first anniversary (a new trend in the wedding industry), this chapter is all about ensuring you look and feel your best when vacationing with your new hubby.

Honeymoon Prep Timeline

As with most things, success is often dependent on serious preparation. Your honeymoon is no exception. Want an extraordinary getaway with your newly betrothed? Start planning well in advance and you'll be fabulously jet-setting when the time comes!

6+ MONTHS BEFORE . . .

- At this point you should, at the very least, know where you'd like to go as well as your budget.

- If you're using a travel agent, start discussing ideas.

- If you need a passport to get to your destination, make sure it is valid for six months after your departure date and have a new one reissued if not.

- Confirm you have necessary visas, if any.

- Book your flights and confirm seat assignments.

- Request special in-flight meals, if desired.

- Start researching hotels.

- Check with a doctor to see if you need any immunizations.

- If you're heading somewhere remote, talk with your doctor about getting a prescription for antibiotics or other hard-to-get medications to travel with in case of emergency.

- Start stocking up on free samples of your favorite beauty products—most freestanding retailers and cosmetics counters in malls will happily give you free travel-size samples, especially if you buy the full size, too . . . and especially if you tell them you're getting married!

3 MONTHS BEFORE . . .

◆ Book hotels and any excursions requiring reservations.

◆ Start reading that guide book so you know what you want to do and see.

◆ Consider getting travel insurance.

◆ Buy luggage if you don't already own it.

◆ If you're on the pill and want to ensure your period doesn't come while away, talk with your gynecologist about possible plans.

1 MONTH BEFORE . . .

◆ Book any must-have dinner reservations. If you're staying at a hotel, the concierge can usually help with this.

◆ Schedule a surprise for your significant other—a couples massage, boat excursion, or romantic dinner are all great options.

◆ Scan the packing list below and make sure you have everything. Buy anything you still need.

◆ Arrange a pet and/or house sitter, if needed.

◆ Reconfirm all your reservations.

2 WEEKS BEFORE . . .

◆ Pack! The next two weeks will be jam packed with all the last-minute things you need to do for the wedding, so get packing out of the way.

◆ Download a new book to read on the plane and/or movies you can watch together.

◆ Plan a hold on newspaper and mail delivery.

◆ Make sure any rent, mortgage payments, or bills due while away are paid ahead of time.

◆ If traveling abroad, consider letting the U.S. State Department know in case of emergency.

◆ Print out travel itineraries if you haven't done so already.

◆ Arrange for a ride to the airport.

24 HOURS BEFORE . . .

- Charge all of your electronics.

- Clean out your fridge of anything that will spoil while you're away.

- Water plants.

- Take out the trash.

- Run the garbage disposal with half a lemon to cut any smells.

- Store valuables.

- Unplug appliances you don't need kept on.

- Set the heat/AC to money-saving mode—or turn them off altogether.

- Lock all windows.

AS YOU'RE LEAVING . . .

- Lock the doors.

- Turn off the lights—or set a timer if you have one.

- Double-check that you have all your travel documents.

- Make sure you have your phone, wallet, and camera.

Traveling Tips: How + What to Pack

Whether you're planning an active adventure or a tranquil escape, there are some packing tips that transcend your location-specific needs (bras and SPF, for example!). Obviously the weight and size of your luggage will be exponentially more cumbersome if you're off on a multi-destination African safari than if you're checking into a luxury resort for the duration of your trip, but nevertheless, these tips will help to ensure you're packed as efficiently as possible, without cutting any corners.

HOW TO PACK + SAVE SPACE

ROLL YOUR CLOTHES. The tighter you roll your clothes, the less room they'll take up and the more room you'll have for other things! Stack them snuggly to save even more space.

GET STUFFING. Stuff socks in your shoes to save space and help your shoes to keep their shape. Pack underwear, bras, and bathing suits in plastic bags, making sure to squeeze out extra air to save room. Bonus: they'll be easier to find, too!

PACK THE MUST-HAVES, NOT THE JUST-IN-CASES. Most of your what-if scenarios will never happen, so don't weigh down your luggage with things you'll likely never need. Heading to the desert? In the off chance it rains, you can buy an umbrella then.

SPLIT UP. Prepare for the worst (and hope for the best) by dividing both of your belongings between two suitcases. That way, if one of your bags is lost, at least you'll each have some of your belongings.

PACK LAYERS, NOT BULK. Thin pieces you can layer will not only be much more versatile, they also take up considerably less room. Even if you're skiing, pack one heavy jacket and otherwise thin layers you can wear underneath.

IF YOU MUST BRING BULKY STUFF, WEAR IT. No need to take up valuable luggage space for those bulky items. Instead, wear your jacket and boots on the plane and save the space for other things instead.

CUT BACK ON SHOES. For most trips, comfortable walking shoes (sneakers, hiking boots, or sandals depending on the terrain), one pair of nice shoes for fancy dinners (that go with all of your evening outfits), and a pair of flip-flops will be more than enough. Sure your pink sundress may look best with your turquoise and pink wedges, but if your gold flats work just as well and go with everything else, pack those instead.

LIMIT YOUR COLOR PALATE. Select your clothes around a similar color palate (with a few pops of color thrown in) and you'll be able to mix and match all of your items to create considerably more outfit options. Pick either black/white/gray or browns/neutrals to start and build from there. Then add in a few lightweight blouses, T-shirts, and/or scarves, in bright hues to give your wardrobe variety.

FOLLOW THE RULES. The last thing you want to do is get to the airport to find out you can't check that third bag of yours. Check your airline's website to ensure everything you're bringing falls within the airline's policies.

WHAT TO PACK

While your needs will vary based on your destination, the length of your trip, and your personal travel style, use this as a jumping off point to ensure you don't forget anything—and look great!

Carry-On Bag Essentials

Pack everything you need to travel, whatever you'll want while on the flight, and anything that's irreplaceable (or at the very least would be a massive inconvenience to have to replace while on your honeymoon).

○ Plane tickets

○ Printed confirmation e-mails for all of your hotels, tours, etc.

○ Drivers' licenses or passports and visas, if required

○ Credit cards, cash, and traveler's checks

○ Copies of your travel arrangements, passports, credit cards and traveler's checks, stored someplace separate from your originals in case they're lost or stolen

○ Emergency phone numbers—include your home, doctor, emergency contacts, dog sitter, and credit card companies

○ Travel insurance information, if applicable

○ Itinerary

○ Prescription medications

○ Contraception, if desired

○ Camera—and an extra memory card

○ Chargers for cell phones, iPads, Kindles, and digital cameras

○ Guidebook

○ Headphones

○ Books, Kindle, playing cards, etc.—things to keep you busy while traveling or lounging poolside

○ A change of clothes, just in case

○ Snacks—if you're traveling internationally, check to see the restrictions on what you're allowed to bring into the country (fruit, nuts, and seeds are often prohibited through customs so make sure you eat them on the plane!)

○ Eye mask, ear plugs, and travel pillow for long flights

○ Headphone splitter—so you can watch the same movie on your iPad or computer with separate headsets

○ Sample sizes of body lotion and face cream—airplanes are dehydrating!

○ Lip balm

○ Sunglasses—even if you're not going somewhere super sunny, you'll be glad to have them. Plus, upon arrival, they brilliantly hide post-flight puffiness.

○ **Tote bag or lightweight backpack to pack everything in**—and that will double as your day bag while away

○ **Any beauty product you both can't live without that meets TSA guidelines** (check all the rest)

HOW TO PACK ANY LIQUID . . .
AND CARRY IT ON BOARD!

1) *Take a large drinking straw and fold just the end onto itself. Secure it with packing tape so the bottom is now closed off and spill-proof.*

2) *Pour or pump your desired liquid into the straw, leave at least ¼ inch empty at the top.*

3) *Fold the top down onto itself and use packing tape to secure.*

4) *Use a permanent marker to label the straw so you know the contents.*

5) *Repeat for each product.*

6) *Toss all of them in a quart-size plastic bag and you're ready to fly!*

7) *If you're traveling to more than one destination, pack tape, too, so you can reseal the straws mid-trip.*

In Your Checked Luggage . . .

This is where the bulk of your stuff should go. If you're checking into a single resort and largely staying put, feel free to go crazy within your airline's bag requirements. If, however, you'll be traveling between destinations or will need to carry your own bags for any portion of your journey, be more mindful of unnecessary weight and, remember, at most destinations you can buy or borrow the worst-case scenario things if you end up needing them.

○ CLOTHES:
Mentally walk through each day of your itinerary and try to pack exactly what you'll *need*, then throw in a few extras that you *want*. Don't forget: underwear, bras, socks, a bathing suit, and a lightweight jacket or sweater.

○ SHOES:
This will depend on your destination, but definitely make sure you have at least one pair of shoes you're comfortable walking in! Wear your bulkiest pair on the plane to save space in your luggage.

○ LINGERIE:
It is your honeymoon, after all.

○ EXTRA DUFFEL BAG:
Pack it in the bottom of your suitcase so you have plenty of room for souvenirs!

○ SMALL PACKETS OF WOOLITE LAUNDRY DETERGENT:
So you can wash a few items in the sink, if necessary

○ BEAUTY PRODUCTS:
Just the necessities

○ HAIR-STYLING TOOLS:
Just the necessities

○ ELECTRICAL CONVERTERS:
If traveling internationally

The Toiletries

Depending on where you're off to (and for how long) you'll need to decide what, if anything, from this list should be brought in your carry-on (per TSA guidelines, of course), what should be checked, and what should be left home altogether because you either don't need it or your hotel provides you with it.

○ **SPF:** If you're traveling to a major city in North America or Europe, it's often easier to buy it when you arrive and not risk a spill in your bag. That being said, if you're traveling someplace remote—or just want to land and lounge poolside—transfer your sunscreen to spill-proof containers for safer travels.

○ **Toothpaste**

○ **Toothbrushes**

○ **Deodorant**

○ **Cotton balls and swabs**—most hotels provide these free of charge, but it's worth checking

○ **Comb/brush**

○ **Hair products and accessories**

○ **Nail file/clippers**

○ **Razors**—and shaving cream if body wash won't do

○ **Contact lenses and solution, if needed**

○ **Shampoo, conditioner, body wash, body lotion**—most hotels provide these so only pack them if you have very sensitive skin or very particular preferences. Or, do like I do, and just pack conditioner (which packs the biggest bang) but make do with the rest.

○ **Hair dryer, curling or straightening iron**

○ **Shower cap**

○ **Face wash, serums, creams, and treatments**—follow the 80/20 rule and only bring the things you're 80 percent likely to need. The rest you'll figure out—or do without!

○ **Extra-virgin cold-pressed coconut oil**—in a small travel container since a little goes a long way.

8 USES FOR COCONUT OIL

Extra-virgin cold-pressed coconut oil isn't merely on my packing list for you because I'm not-so-secretly obsessed with it, but also because it's the most multi-use beauty product I own, allowing you to pack less without compromising results. Don't believe me? Here are eight ways you can use it on your honeymoon alone.

1) **Remove waterproof eye makeup.** *Gently rub coconut oil over eye makeup and use a cotton round to remove both the oil and the makeup. Repeat until the cotton round is clean. Leave residue to moisturize the gentle eye area.*

2) **Banish blemishes.** *After cleansing, apply a small amount of antibacterial coconut oil to your face to curb sebum production and fight acne. Your body will think your skin has all the oil it needs and stop producing the pore-clogging kind of oil while simultaneously fighting the bacteria on the surface of your skin.*

3) **Fight fine lines.** *Use coconut oil as an anti-aging face and eye cream to fight fine lines with its hydrating and exfoliating properties.*

4) **Banish behind-the-arm bumps.** *If you suffer from small white or red bumps on the backs of your arms, apply coconut oil twice a day. The lauric acid will help to gently exfoliate them away.*

5) **Get a closer shave.** *Apply coconut oil to dry legs, underarms, or bikini line before getting in the shower or bath. Shave, as usual.*

6) **Scrub away dull skin.** *Mix two tablespoons of coconut oil with ¼ cup sugar (you can even nab some free sugar packets at breakfast!) to create the perfect exfoliating scrub.*

7) **Soothe sunburned skin.** *Scorched by the sun's rays? Apply coconut oil to burned skin to soothe discomfort, prevent peeling, fight infection, and encourage faster cell turnover.*

8) **Whiten teeth.** *Vigorously swish a tablespoon of coconut oil in your mouth for ten minutes before spitting out to break down plaque and whiten your teeth.*

Makeup Must-Haves

You'll be taking lots of pictures and want to look your best, but you don't want to carry (or deal with!) a load of cosmetics. Bring these products, though, and you'll neither compromise results nor convenience.

○ **TINTED MOISTURIZER WITH SPF:** It evens out your skin tone and gives you a baseline sunscreen, too.

○ **CONCEALER:** The stress of wedding planning and subsequent release when it's all down, can wreak havoc on your skin (not even to mention the under eye circles you may start your trip with from dancing all night).

○ **LIP + CHEEK BALM:** That can double as your blush and lipstick

○ **EYELASH CURLER:** For the look of mascara, without the risk of it running down your face

○ **WATERPROOF MASCARA**

○ **LUMINIZER:** To add just a pop of brightness to your collarbones, cheekbones, and eyes

○ **BRONZER:** Especially if you may need to correct unintended tan lines

○ **POWDER:** If you tend to get oily, or you're traveling someplace humid, it will help stop shine.

Makeup Maybes

○ **EYELINER**

○ **ADDITIONAL LIP GLOSSES AND LIPSTICKS**

○ **EYE SHADOW:** Pick one neutral palette hue you can wear day and night

For Emergencies

Just as you needed a Bridal Survival Kit for your wedding day, you similarly should have one packed for your honeymoon. Depending on your destination, your specific needs will vary, but use this as a guide to ensure the best possible time without any unintended hitches. If you'll be able to easily procure these at your destination, though, feel free to just buy them there, if needed.

○ TAMPONS/PADS: Stress and hormones can mess with even the most predictable of cycles, so better to be safe.

○ ANTACID + DIARRHEA MEDICINE: Eating most of your meals out will put you at increased risk for questionable ingredients (especially if you're traveling internationally). Be prepared just in case whatever you're eating doesn't sit well.

○ ANTIHISTAMINES: Just in case allergies kick in while in a new environment.

○ MOTION SICKNESS MEDICINE: Especially if you're planning excursions.

○ PAIN RELIEVER: Whether you're lounging beachside or hiking Machu Picchu, pack a general over-the-counter pain reliever to help relieve everything from the discomfort of a sunburn to the pain of a sprained ankle.

○ BAND-AIDS: Pack a variety, including blister-specific ones. Take them out of the box to save space.

○ CORTISONE CREAM

○ ANTIBIOTIC OINTMENT

○ ANTIBACTERIAL WIPES

Handy Extras

○ ZIPLOC BAGS:
To store wet swimsuits or protect your camera if it rains

○ SEWING KIT

○ STAIN-REMOVING PENS

○ SMALL BACKPACK(S):
For day excursions

○ OLD SNEAKERS:
A pair that you can leave behind if they get ruined

○ WORKOUT CLOTHES:
If you plan on hitting the gym or running outdoors (a great way to explore a new place and stay fit!)

○ COMPACT UMBRELLA OR RAIN PONCHOS:
Only if there is an 80 percent chance you'll need it—otherwise, you can always borrow or buy one there

○ INSECT REPELLENT AND ANTI-ITCH SPRAY

○ HAT

○ MASSAGE OIL

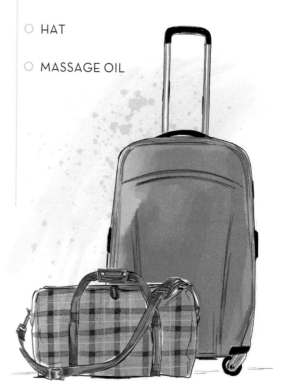

WHAT TO LEAVE BEHIND
WITH FAMILY OR FRIENDS

◆ *Your itinerary and hotel phone numbers*

◆ *Photocopies of your passport, credit cards, and traveler's check receipts*

◆ *A sealed envelope with a copy of your wills, life insurance-policy numbers, and pertinent financial info*

◆ *Your computer. Now's the time to focus on you and disconnect. No work allowed!*

◆ *Depending on your destination and planned activities, consider leaving your engagement and wedding rings at home so they're safe. Otherwise, make sure to confirm with your hotel that there is a safe for you to use if you go scuba diving or hiking.*

Planes, Trains, + Automobiles: Transportation-Specific Tips

IF YOU'RE TRAVELING BY PLANE . . .

◆ Always travel with a clean face. Arriving fresh-faced is better than arriving clogged and dull!

◆ Moisturize before takeoff and every three hours thereafter until you land. Don't forget about your hands, too.

◆ If you're flying during the day, don't forget to apply sunscreen.

◆ Drink at least one cup of water for every hour you're in the air. Airplanes are desperately dehydrating!

◆ Cleanse your skin when you arrive to remove the dirt and grime of the airplane.

IF YOU'RE TRAVELING BY CAR . . .

◆ Apply sunscreen: Don't forget the backs of your hands—and reapply every two hours.

◆ Wear a hat and sunglasses if it's especially sunny to protect your skin from sun damage.

◆ Bring enough water to ensure you stay hydrated for the duration of the ride.

◆ If driving through heavily polluted or dusty areas, put your car's air filter on "internal" so it recirculates the clean air inside instead of pulling the polluted air from outside in.

The Honeymoon Diet

You're on vacation and want to indulge. I get it. But the last thing you want to do is spend your honeymoon bloated and feeling gross. If you have a significant amount of time between your wedding and honeymoon and have already reintroduced your favorite foods into your diet (as per Chapter 2) and are feeling great, keep doing what you're doing! If, however, you are feeling anything shy of amazing, turn back to page 36 and get down and dirty with your food journal, cutting out anything standing in your way from feeling like the radiant bride you are. Alternatively, if you're off on your honeymoon immediately following your nuptials, it's to your advantage to stick with your current diet (wherever you are in the process) and hold off on indulging, lest you end up with a stomachache or erupting skin while on your honeymoon.

That being said, if you can't resist a big bowl of creamy pasta in Italy or a sugar-packed margarita in Mexico, here's what you need to know.

GO SLOW

Start with a small portion of anything you haven't eaten in the last six weeks and see how you feel twenty-four hours later before slowly working your way up to a full-size portion.

CHEW THOROUGHLY

Make sure you chew slowly and thoroughly to help your body digest your food most efficiently. Your stomach doesn't have teeth, so it needs to work considerably harder to break down food that's not properly pulverized. Chew properly and you'll be far less likely to feel the effects of a sudden gluten binge. You'll also be less gassy.

PREVENT WITH PROBIOTICS

If you're planning on indulging the second you say "I do" and there's nothing I can do to convince you otherwise, make sure to take a daily probiotic to balance out your belly's good bacteria to ensure your stomach is in the best shape possible for handling whatever you throw its way.

TAKE DIGESTIVE ENZYMES

If you know you're about to throw caution to the wind, take a digestive enzyme (I like Dr. Frank Lipman's plant-based ones) with the first bite to help your body break down proteins, carbohydrates, and fats both for better absorption and less bloating and gas.

WEAR LINGERIE

Not only because you'll be having a lot of sexy time, but also because it will help you *feel* sexy and in tune with your body, which will help you to naturally and easily feed your body exactly what it needs—and, yes, what it wants—all without overindulging.

14 Ways to Ban Belly Bloat

———◇———

Traveling seems to have a way of messing with our digestive tracts. Sure, it's partly because you're eating many of your meals out and, thus, giving up a bit of control over your diet, but it's also the result of merely switching our routines, which causes internal stress (even if you finally feel far from stressed, you may even say relaxed!). If there is a time you'd like to avoid bloating and constipation at all costs, though, it's probably your honeymoon! Thankfully, you're not destined to feel or look bloated with these tips.

1) CUT CARBONATION (YES, EVEN CHAMPAGNE). Those bubbles have to go some-where . . . and you don't want them in your belly! Sure, a champagne toast seems romantic, but wine is a far better choice for keeping you looking and feeling like your sexiest self.

2) DRINK MORE WATER. A lot of people think that if their bodies are retaining water, they should cut back, but the opposite is actually the case. Your body is holding on to fluids for fear of dehydration. Flush your body with water, though, and your body will let the excess go.

3) SAYONARA STRAWS. Whatever you're drinking, drink it from the glass and not with a straw so you don't inadvertently swallow air.

4) SAY "NO" TO SALT. The salt shaker may be calling your name, but it's also calling that water you're drinking and holding on to it for dear life.

5) COOK YOUR VEGGIES. When vegetables are cooked, the fiber structure is broken down, making them easier for your body to digest. Raw veggies, on the other hand, (especially cruci-ferous ones like broccoli, brussels sprouts, cabbage, and cauliflower) cause excess gas as your body works to break them down.

6) RELISH ROSEMARY. Spot rosemary roasted vegetables on the menu? Order away! The flavorful herb helps to fight gas and inflammation. You can steep some in hot water for a bloat-banishing tonic, too!

7) ADD FERMENTED VEGETABLES TO YOUR DIET. Kimchi, sauerkraut, and other fermented vegetables are packed with digestion-aiding probiotics. Plus, they're loaded with flavor. Just be sure to balance them with plenty of water since they're often high in sodium.

8) PACK IN THE POTASSIUM. The mineral helps to regulate sodium and fluids in your body, keeping bloating at bay. Sweet potatoes, bananas, tomatoes, clams, and prunes are all great choices.

9) SKIP THE GUM. You may think of it as an easy way to fix that oral craving without overindulging, but while you may not be swallowing the gum, you are swallowing loads of air and belly-bloating artificial sugars with each chew.

10) AVOID FAUX SUGARS. Your body doesn't know how to process faux sugars and sugar alcohols (like xylitol, sorbitol, or maltitol), resulting (for many people) in gas, bloating, and sometimes even diarrhea!

11) CUT ACIDS. Coffee, citrus fruit, and spicy foods can all increase the acid in your GI tract, leaving it irritated and inflamed.

12) ADD ASPARAGUS. It may make your pee smell, but it's a natural diuretic, helping your body to flush retained fluids away.

13) MASSAGE YOUR STOMACH. This may sound weird, but some gentle massage in the direction your body naturally digests helps to move your GI tract along. Start at your right hip, move up toward your sternum, and then down to your left hip in a clockwise motion.

14) GET MOVING. If you're constipated or retaining fluids, moving the outside of your body helps to move things along inside your body as well. Just a fifteen-minute brisk walk will do the trick.

Your Honeymoon Beauty Routine

You've been taking your beauty routine so seriously up until your wedding day and there's no reason to switch up the routine that's been working for you now. But pay attention to where you're traveling (especially the temperature and humidity) and adjust accordingly. Heading to the desert? Make sure you moisturize more than you do at home. Off to a humid beach? Pack all the products you'll need to ensure your hair isn't a frizz-fest. Otherwise, keep it simple and let your beauty radiate from within.

Need help feeling just a bit sexier?

◆ Pack different lingerie for each day and reveal a new ensemble each night you're away.

◆ Put together a sexy playlist (Marvin Gaye and Sade, anyone?).

◆ Do something active. Nothing gets your adrenaline going—and makes you feel sexy!—more than doing something that gets your blood pumping. No, you don't need to hit the gym together (unless you want to!); you can go for a romantic hike, try kayaking, or give a local dance class a try.

And, finally, remember this is the time to celebrate your relationship, relish in your newly wedded status, and enjoy each other wholeheartedly. Have fun, relax, savor—and don't let crummy weather, the wrong shoes, or bad hair days take away from any of it.

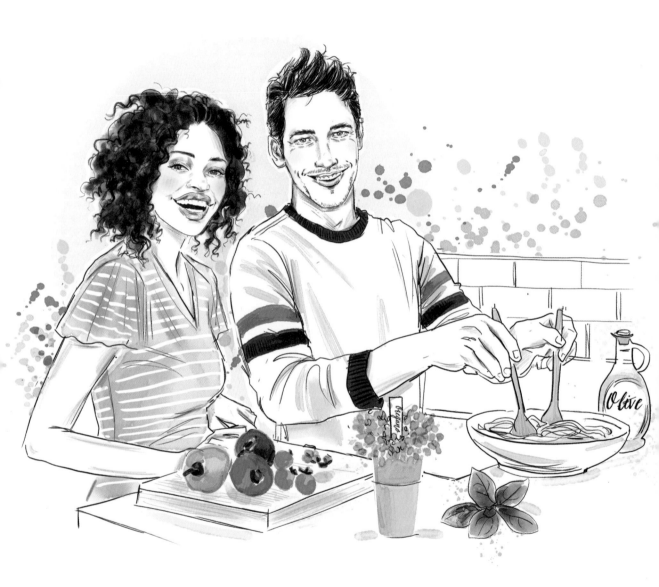

LIVING HAPPILY EVER AFTER: THE RADIANT WIFE

FROM THE MOMENT THAT RING was slipped on your finger you've been preparing for your happily ever after, and here you are! You thrived (or at least survived) from saying "yes" to saying "I do," and now it is time to embark on your blissfully married life. Some say this is the point where the work really begins, and I'm no relationship expert so perhaps they're right, but when it comes to beauty and wellness, that's a piece of vegan, gluten-free cake. And since I'm pretty sure that a happy, healthy wife is at least half of every happy, healthy marriage, you're probably off to a great start!

So how do we maintain our health and happiness and continue to radiate anniversary after anniversary? We keep prioritizing both ourselves and our partners. We take care of ourselves, inside and out. We listen to our bodies. We treat ourselves with the same love and respect we expect from others. We eat well. We exercise. We pamper. We transition from being a Radiant Bride to a Radiant Wife. Here's how!

Beauty Beyond the Big Day

Your wedding day and honeymoon may be over, but that is no reason to undo all our progress. Instead, keep up with everything you have learned! A thorough skincare routine should never stop, only be reassessed and perhaps elevated over time. At least twice a year, reevaluate any face makeup shades (your skin tone likely changes at least one shade between summer and winter) and adjust your foundation, concealer, blush, and bronzer accordingly. The more the climate in your city changes over the course of the year, the more your skincare products will have to vary as well, with more hydration in the drier, cooler months and more oil-free products in the more humid, hotter months.

One of the biggest mistakes I see women make is to do a serious clean out and restock (like the one in Chapter 6) and then never do it again, even though our skin is constantly changing. While you should be regularly cleaning out and restocking your makeup and skincare according to the expiration schedule on page 108, it's equally essential to do a biyearly check in with your skin to address changes in tone and texture and to modify your skincare products and makeup accordingly. Noticing more fine lines and wrinkles? Up the ante on your retinol routine. A stressful new job leaving you with under-eye circles? Look for an eye cream with caffeine in it and keep it in the fridge. Skin showing signs of hyperpigmentation or otherwise uneven tone? Maybe it's time to add a tinted moisturizer or foundation to your daily routine and to take your sunscreen to the next level. Unless you make it a point to evaluate your complexion regularly, it's easy not to see the changes at all (or at least not until it's well past the earliest signs, when all skincare concerns are more easily addressed).

How to Look + Feel Your Best Anniversary After Anniversary

Most brides throw caution to the wind (with their diets, anyway!) the second they say "I do." You, though, my magnificent Mrs., know better. And while I know I've made it crystal clear why you shouldn't drop all the great habits you've adopted, that doesn't mean you have to—or should—remain on the Radiant Bride Diet forever.

If there are still some foods you're avoiding on the detox plan and you're ready to try to reintroduce them, turn back to page 42 and follow the same guidelines we used to reintroduce foods after your twenty-one-day Radiant Bride Detox. Just because you're no longer worried about fitting into the most expensive dress you've ever owned doesn't mean you should just throw all your hard work to the wind and dive head first into an extra-large pepperoni pizza—especially since the goal here is looking and feeling radiant, not merely thin. By taking your time and conscientiously reintroducing foods you have yet to add back into your diet, you'll learn more about how foods react in your body and how you should continue to eat regularly in order to look and, more important, feel radiant always!

If, however, you're feeling better than ever, feel free to stick with your current eating plan for as long you like, with a couple of additional rules:

1) CONTINUE TO LISTEN TO YOUR BODY. Remember: our bodies are constantly changing (during our monthly cycles, throughout the changing seasons, and over the years), so it's essential to regularly reevaluate your personalized diet. For most of us, it's a good idea to repeat the twenty-one-day detox at least once a year to see if your immune response to food has changed at all. (Perhaps a new yearly New Year's resolution?!) At least continue to look for patterns between what you eat and how you feel and to adjust your diet accordingly if any negative patterns emerge.

2) BE FLEXIBLE. The only successful diets are those that provide for flexibility and fun, without guilt. Sure, willpower is great, but no one wants to rely on that alone—or feel guilty when it fails you (because it probably will). Instead, I want you to give yourself permission to eat anything you want, whenever you want, so long as it's mindfully savored. Like a little kid who's told not to do something and then immediately is overcome by an unbreakable desire to do just that, as adults we do the same thing when we're told we can't eat something. We become overcome by cravings. Instead of trying to fight them (and feeling guilty if we succumb), give yourself permission to indulge. But, when you do, don't stand guilty in the kitchen shoving your face while no one is looking. Instead, make yourself a plate, sit down, and take a deep breath before you start eating. Chew thoroughly, swallow mindfully. Enjoy it fully. And don't ever, ever, ever feel guilty (it does nothing other than raise your stress hormones!).

Post-nuptial Fitness

You no longer need a fitness routine catered to your dress, but you most definitely still need a fitness routine if for no other reason than you heart health. Heart disease is the number-one killer of women, making it more deadly than all forms of cancer. One of the best ways to help keep that ticker of yours ticking is to keep your body moving.

The American Heart Association recommends forty minutes of moderate to vigorous aerobic exercise three to four times a week and strength training at least twice per week, so let's make that the goal. More than just keeping your heart beating, cardio and strength training also help to increase your metabolism, increase your muscular and bone strength, reduce your risk of injury, pump you full of mood-boosting endorphins, and more. Hopefully, at this point, you've found some form of exercise you like and can continue to do that. If not, keep trying new ways to keep moving and remember, you don't need to hit the gym to exercise. House cleaning, a brisk walk with your dog, rollerblading with girlfriends, and even sex, all can count as exercise, too!

Need help staying motivated? Turn back to page 57 for tips.

You: Happily Ever After

———◇———

Your wedding day may have been the happiest day of your life, but your marriage will not make you happy. Instead, a happy marriage is dependent on first being a happy person. So, how do you ensure your own happiness?

BE KIND TO YOUR BODY AND MIND. Treat your body with the same love and respect you treat others. Let go of judgments and criticisms. You wouldn't stand in front of your best friend and tell her all the things you likely say to yourself in the mirror, so don't say them to yourself, either.

FORGIVE YOURSELF. As women, we are far too hard on ourselves. Forgive and let go.

SAVOR SUNSHINE. Even just five minutes outside makes everyone happier.

EXERCISE. If for no other reason than the endorphin boost, get moving. It will also help you to appreciate your body more.

PRIORITIZE YOURSELF. It can be easy to lose yourself in your relationships to others—as a daughter, wife, mother, employee, and more. But you can only help others if you take care of yourself first. Make sure you follow the airplane adage to "put the oxygen mask on yourself before helping others" and you'll not only feel better about yourself, you'll also show up better in all of those roles. To piggyback off of that, don't be afraid to schedule "me time" where you can explore new hobbies, dive into a book, or hang out with girlfriends.

SLEEP. Everyone's a bit unhappy when overtired! Aim for eight hours of sleep and you'll look and feel better.

GIVE COMPLIMENTS + WRITE THANK-YOU NOTES. It's amazing how much happiness you can get from putting a smile on someone else's face. Try it!

SPEND TIME WITH FRIENDS. Friendships are essential to our happiness, but they need nurturing. Even when you're swamped and stressed, shoot off a quick text or e-mail to a friend asking how she is or plan to call your best bud from college on your commute.

APPRECIATE WHAT YOU HAVE. It can be easy to find yourself in a "grass is always greener" rut, which makes you nothing short of miserable. Instead, every day write down five things that you're grateful for. It's amazing how many more will come to you once you open your eyes to this exercise.

Happily Ever After in Your Marriage

The most blissfully in-love, married-forever couples know some things the rest of us merely hope to figure out. But that's a mistake. You wouldn't hope to figure out how to drive by trial and error; you would get advice from someone who has been doing it well for some time. Do the same with regard to your relationships. Especially since there really isn't any room for the error part in a marriage. Here are some lessons shared with me by some of the happiest, most blissfully married people I know. They may just help you, too.

PLAN DATE NIGHTS. You may be living together, but that doesn't mean you're spending quality time together. Plan regular date nights, get dressed up, don't talk about household chores (or kids, if you have them). Just be together and connect.

SAY "I LOVE YOU" BEFORE BED. Even if you're still a little bit angry over something.

HAVE MORE SEX. It's normal for desire to waiver over time. Do it anyway. Studies show that having sex doesn't merely beget more sex, it also improves the mood of both partners, diminishes feelings of anger (it's why makeup sex is so important). Plus, the physical connection leads to greater feelings of emotional connection.

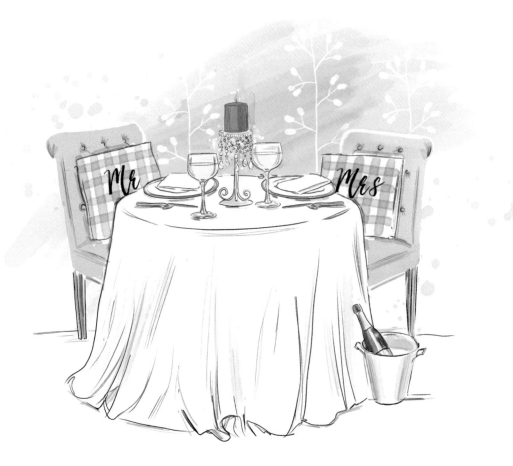

TRY NEW THINGS. When your routine is in a rut, your marriage won't be far behind. Make a list of new things you've always wanted to try and do them together. The excitement of doing something new (bonus points if it's adrenaline-pumping) will bring you closer together.

HAVE SEPARATE FRIENDS. Your marriage should be your closest relationship, but not your only one. Desire is dependent on distance, so make sure you spend some time apart (although not too much!).

PHYSICALLY CONNECT EVERY DAY. Hold hands, kiss, grab butts. Even if it's just for a few seconds, it will help keep you physically connected.

BE NICE. It may sound obvious, but being critical and nitpicky is one of the quickest ways to problems in relationships. And no, you can't just balance your criticism with a compliment. In fact, studies show it takes approximately five positive statements to outweigh a single negative one. Keep that in mind the next time you feel the need to say something negative to your partner!

TREAT YOUR SPOUSE LIKE YOU DID WHEN YOU FIRST STARTED DATING. Sounds easy enough, but in practice it's harder than you may think. When you first started dating, though, you wouldn't be thirty minutes late to dinner or roll your eyes when asked to take out the trash, so don't do it now that you're married, either.

GO TO BED AT THE SAME TIME. Getting into bed at the same time for some quality time is a great way to end the day on a positive, connected note. Have different schedules that require different bedtimes? When the first-to-bed partner is ready to hit the sack, both partners should climb in and get cozy, even if it's just for a few minutes of cuddling before the awake partner goes and watches TV.

BE OPEN AND HONEST ABOUT YOUR WANTS AND NEEDS. Not feeling connected? Feeling frustrated? Don't let feelings of angst fester. Talk them out. Your partner isn't a mind reader!

FORGIVE FAST. Holding a grudge doesn't serve anyone—and most definitely doesn't serve your relationship. Say sorry. Accept apologies. Move on.

THINK SMALL. Grand gestures are always nice, but it's the small, regular stuff that actually makes a difference. Offer to do the dishes (even when it's not your night), write a love note, and give lots of compliments.

LAUGH OFTEN. Couples that laugh together, stay together.

PUT YOUR PARTNER FIRST. A stressful job or (more stressful) kids may rule your schedule, but they shouldn't wedge their way between you and your partner. My incredible parents have always (now for fifty-plus years!) been a steadfast team, always putting each other first.

BE FRIENDS. Being lovers and roommates is nice, but it's definitely not enough—you need to be friends, too.

GIVE COMPLIMENTS. Every day, try to think of something you're grateful for about your partner and share it—it will make both of you appreciate how lucky you are.

Cheers to your radiantly happily ever after!

Index

Acknowledgments

MY HEART IS BURSTING WITH GRATITUDE FOR . . .

My family—especially Mom and Dad who consistently show me the power of love, the possibilities in marriage, and the value of family.

Cindy De La Hoz, Susan Van Horn, and the rest of the team at Running Press—thank you for believing in me. Again!

Tracy Turnbull—I am so appreciative of your hard work in bringing my vision to life!

Michele Martin—I couldn't have done any of this without your support and guidance. I am eternally grateful.

CAA—especially Becky Sendrow, Stephanie Paciullo, Ali Spiesman, and Jordan Solomon. I am humbled by your belief in me and thankful for all you do to support my mission to help all women look and feel their best.

Coded PR—in particular, Jennifer Wilson and Jennifer Jimenez—I don't know how you do it, but you always do!

My friends who I have seen walk down the aisle, or one day will—you are all *RADIANT* exactly as you are.

My Beauty Bean-ers—from the talented writers who contribute, to the beauties who visit the site daily, this wouldn't be possible without you.

Love always,
Alexis